100

Best Health
Foods

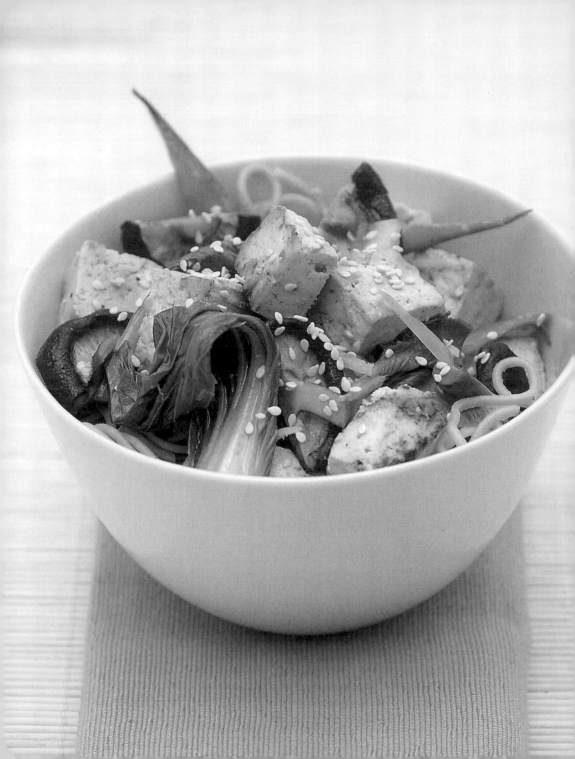

100
Best Health
Foods

The ultimate superfoods for healthy living including 100 nutritious recipes

This edition published in 2010
LOVE FOOD is an imprint of Parragon Books Ltd

Parragon
Queen Street House
4 Queen Street
Bath BA1 1HE, UK

ISBN: 978-1-4075-6445-6

Printed in China

Created and produced by Ivy Contract
Consultant: Judith Wills
New photography by Clive Streeter

Notes for the Reader
This book uses imperial, metric, and US cup measurements. Follow the
same units of measurement throughout; do not mix imperial and metric.
All spoon measurements are level: teaspoons are assumed to be 5 ml,
and tablespoons are assumed to be 15 ml. Unless otherwise stated,
milk is assumed to be whole, eggs and individual vegetables, such as
potatoes, are medium, and pepper is freshly ground black pepper.

The times given are an approximate guide only. Preparation times differ
according to the techniques used by different people and the cooking
times may also vary from those given as a result of the type of oven used.
Optional ingredients, variations, or serving suggestions have not been
included in the calculations.

Recipes using raw or very lightly cooked eggs should be avoided by
infants, the elderly, pregnant women, convalescents, and anyone with
a chronic condition. Pregnant and breastfeeding women are advised to
avoid eating peanuts and peanut products, smoked or cured meats and
fish, and unpasteurized dairy products. People with nut allergies should
be aware that some of the store-bought ingredients used in the recipes in
this book may contain nuts. Always check the packaging before use.

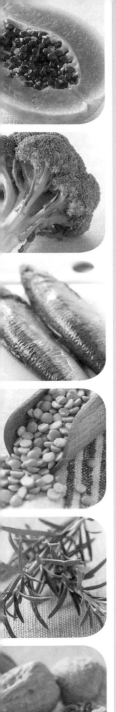

CONTENTS

INTRODUCTION

We all want to eat well—and *100 Best Health Foods* is the book for everyone who wants to know which foods really are the healthiest in the world and why.

Today most of us understand the importance of providing good, healthy meals for ourselves and our families. Healthy eating helps our children grow and thrive, developing strong bodies. Health foods can boost our own immune system and offer protection from cancers, diabetes, and cardiovascular disease. Most noticeably, a good diet helps our bodies run smoothly throughout the day—it improves our brain function, increases our energy levels, and helps us relax and sleep well.

What is a health food?

With a constant stream of conflicting information, sometimes it can be hard to know what foods really do form a healthy diet. This book examines foods that have a proven track record in enhancing health or offering protection from diseases. For each of the foods, the positive health benefits have been well-established and confirmed in trials across the world over a period of years.

Our definition of a health food is one that has a higher-than-average content of the important, and sometimes hard to get, vitamins and minerals, or an equally good range of the plant chemicals and other recently discovered nutrient-like compounds that studies have shown to have major health impacts. These will

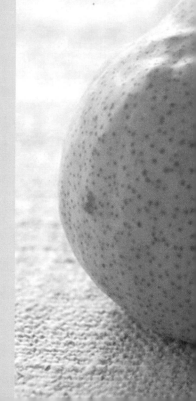

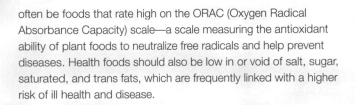

often be foods that rate high on the ORAC (Oxygen Radical Absorbance Capacity) scale—a scale measuring the antioxidant ability of plant foods to neutralize free radicals and help prevent diseases. Health foods should also be low in or void of salt, sugar, saturated, and trans fats, which are frequently linked with a higher risk of ill health and disease.

The importance of a varied diet

A list of only one hundred foods cannot be definitive and there are many more foods that are healthy and nutritious in their own right, but didn't quite make this list. If your own favorite vegetable, fruit, grain, or other food isn't listed, that doesn't mean it won't add positive nutrition to your overall diet.

A healthy diet for most people is one that includes 5–7 portions of vegetables and fruits a day (a good balance is 3–4 vegetables and 2–3 fruits, 2–3 portions of whole grains such as whole grain barley, brown rice, and oats, and 2–3 portions of lean protein such as skinless chicken, lowfat plain yogurt, lentils, or crab. Your diet should also include regular amounts of oily fish, nuts and seeds, plant oils, herbs, and spices.

Remember, no one food can make you healthy on its own—aim instead for a varied and balanced diet. This means trying to include many of the foods in this book into your diet on a regular basis, and varying your choices daily. The diverse set of recipes included in this book offers ways to combine several foods featured and provide a wide range of meals with ideas you can enjoy throughout the day—from breakfast to dessert.

The information in *100 Best Health Foods* will help you build your own perfect diet and, just as importantly, you will enjoy learning more about the wonderful world of healthy, natural foods.

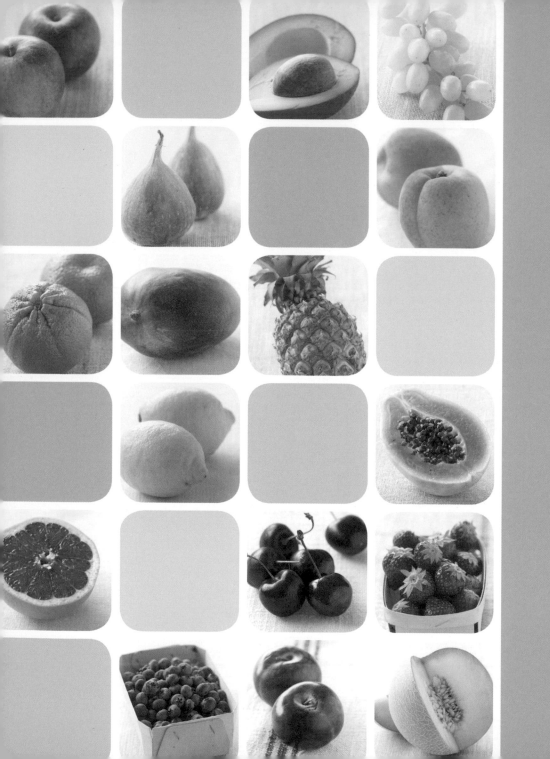

FRUITS

Rich in vitamin C, antioxidants, and fiber, fruits offer a wide range of health benefits. They are also a great source of energy. Fruits can be added to almost any meal or eaten as a healthy snack throughout the day.

(V) Suitable for vegetarians

(D) Ideal for dieters

(P) Suitable for pregnancy

(C) Suitable for children over 5 years

(Q) Quick to prepare and cook

01

APPLES

In recent years, scientific evidence has shown that the old proverb, "An apple a day keeps the doctor away," may be correct.

Although apples don't, with the exception of potassium, contain any particular vitamin or mineral, they do contain high levels of various plant chemicals, including the flavonoid quercetin, which has anticancer and anti-inflammatory action. They are also a valuable source of pectin, a soluble fiber that can help lower "bad" cholesterol and help prevent colon cancer. Research has found that adults who eat apples have smaller waistlines, less abdominal fat, and lower blood pressure than those who don't—apples may also prevent asthma in children. Apples are also virtually fat-free.

- Rich in flavonoids for healthy heart and lungs.
- Ideal snack for dieters as they are low in calories, low on the glycemic index (GI), and can keep hunger at bay.
- Fiber content is rich in pectin, which can improve the blood lipids profile and reduce "bad" cholesterol.
- A good source of potassium, which can prevent fluid retention.

Practical tips:
Don't keep your apples in a light, hot room as they will rapidly lose their vitamin C content. Instead, keep them in a plastic bag with air holes in the refrigerator, or in a cool, dark cupboard. Try to eat the skin as it contains up to five times as many plant chemicals as the flesh. When preparing apples, put the cut slices into a bowl of water with 1–2 tablespoons of lemon juice to prevent browning.

DID YOU KNOW?

Research has found a link between quercetin—found in apples—and protection against Alzheimer's disease.

MAJOR NUTRIENTS PER AVERAGE-SIZED APPLE

Kcalories	60
Total fat	Trace
Protein	Trace
Carbohydrate	16 g
Fiber	2.8 g
Vitamin C	5 mg
Potassium	123 mg

Stuffed baked apples

SERVES 4

2½ heaping tbsp blanched
　almonds
⅓ cup plumped dried apricots
1 piece preserved ginger, drained
1 tbsp honey
1 tbsp syrup from the preserved
　ginger jar
4 tbsp rolled oats
4 large baking apples

Method

1 Preheat the oven to
350°F/180°C. Using a sharp
knife, chop the almonds,
apricots, and preserved
ginger very finely. Set aside
until needed.

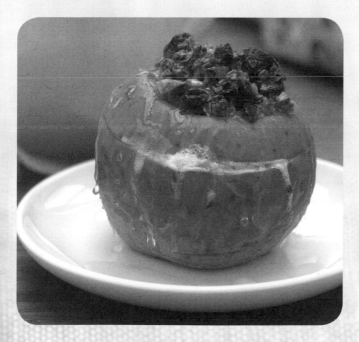

2 Place the honey and syrup in
a saucepan and heat until the
honey has melted. Stir in the
oats and cook gently over
low heat for 2 minutes.
Remove the saucepan
from the heat and stir in
the almonds, apricots, and
preserved ginger.

3 Core the apples, widen
the tops slightly, and score
horizontally around the
circumference of each to
prevent the skins bursting
during cooking. Place the
apples in an ovenproof dish
and fill the cavities with the
stuffing. Pour just enough
water into the dish to come
about one-third of the way
up the apples. Bake in
the preheated oven for 40
minutes, or until tender.
Serve immediately.

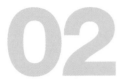

02

AVOCADOS

The avocado is a rich source of monounsaturated fats for heart health and is packed with important nutrients.

Avocados are very high in fat, but this fat is mostly mono-unsaturated. The oleic acid contained in monounsaturates can lower the risk of breast cancer, and monounsaturates can help to reduce "bad" blood cholesterol levels. Avocados also have a large range of nutrients, including vitamins C, E, and B6, folate, iron, magnesium, and potassium, and antioxidant plant chemicals beta-sitosterol, which can also help lower blood cholesterol, and glutathione, which protects against cancer.

DID YOU KNOW?

Extra virgin avocado oil is now widely available—use it for roasting, drizzling over salads, or serve it as a dip with crusty bread.

- High vitamin E content boosts the immune system, keeps skin healthy, and helps prevent heart disease.
- Lutein content helps protect against eye cataracts and macular degeneration.
- High monounsaturated fat content helps lower cholesterol.
- Good source of magnesium for a healthy heart.

Practical tips:

Choose avocados that have unblemished skins without soft spots, which suggest bruising. They're ready to eat if the flesh yields slightly when pressed with the thumb. To hasten ripening, put them in a paper bag with a banana. To prepare, cut lengthwise down to the pit and twist to separate the two halves. Pierce the pit with the tip of a knife, then pull the pit out. Once cut, use lemon juice, vinegar, or vinaigrette dressing, to avoid discoloration.

MAJOR NUTRIENTS PER AVERAGE-SIZED AVOCADO

Kcalories	240
Total fat	3 g
Protein	22 g
Carbohydrate	12.8 g
Fiber	5 g
Vitamin C	9 mg
Potassium	728 mg
Vitamin E	3 mg

Spicy avocado dip

SERVES 4

2 large avocados
juice of 1–2 limes
2 large garlic cloves, crushed
1 tsp mild chili powder,
   or to taste
salt and pepper

Method

1 Cut the avocados in half. Remove the pits and skin and discard.
2 Place the avocado flesh in a food processor with the juice of 1 or 2 limes, according to taste. Add the garlic and chili powder and process until smooth.
3 Transfer to a large serving bowl, season to taste, and serve.

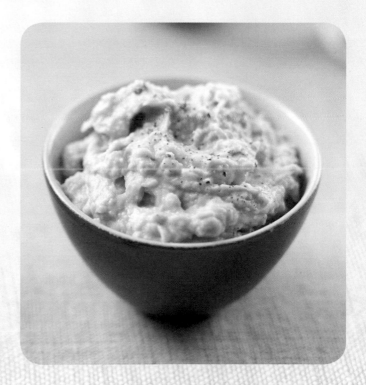

03

GRAPES

Grapes are rich in polyphenols—which protect our hearts, improve circulation, and help lower cholesterol—and have antifungal properties.

All grape varieties contain beneficial compounds, mainly polyphenols, and most of these are found in the skin. Black, purple, and red varieties also contain much higher levels of the flavonoid quercetin and anthocyanins—the dark pigments—and both may help prevent cancer, heart, and cardiovascular disease. The antioxidant benefits of paler-colored grapes are mainly from their catechin content. Resveratrol, another antioxidant present in all grapes, has been linked to the prevention or inhibition of cancer and heart disease, degenerative nerve disease, and viral infections, and may also be linked to protection against Alzheimer's disease.

- Rich source of polyphenols, for cancer prevention and a healthy cardiovascular system.
- Quercetin can improve blood cholesterol profile and has an anticlotting action.
- Antiviral and antifungal action.
- Good source of vitamin C.

Practical tips:
Wash grapes before use—they may have been sprayed with pesticides—and store in the refrigerator or a cool room to preserve vitamin C content and prevent deterioration. If using in a dessert, cut at the last minute to prevent the cut side from browning.

DID YOU KNOW?

Over 70 percent of world grape production is used for wine, 27 percent is for fresh fruit, and 2 percent for dried fruit.

MAJOR NUTRIENTS PER 3½ oz/100 g GRAPES

Kcalories	70
Total fat	Trace
Protein	0.7 g
Carbohydrate	18 g
Fiber	0.9 g
Vitamin C	10.8 mg
Potassium	191 mg

White grape and lemon foam

SERVES 2

*scant 1 cup white grapes,
seeded or seedless, plus
extra to serve*

*generous ¾ cup sparkling
mineral water*

*2 large scoops of frozen
plain yogurt*

*1½ tbsp concentrated
frozen lemonade*

Method

1 Place the grapes, mineral water, frozen yogurt, and lemonade in a food processor and process until smooth.

2 Pour the foam into glasses, top with a few grapes, and serve.

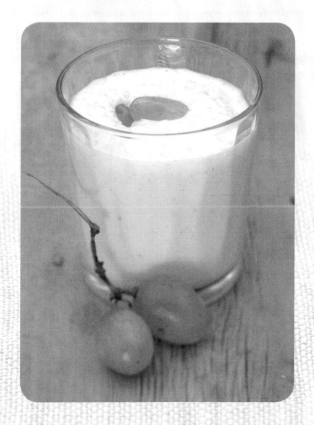

04

DID YOU KNOW?

The leaves of the fig tree are edible. Fig-leaf liquid extract has antidiabetic properties, reducing the amount of insulin needed by some people with diabetes.

MAJOR NUTRIENTS PER FRESH FIG

Kcalories	47
Total fat	Trace
Protein	0.5 g
Carbohydrate	12.3 g
Fiber	1.9 g
Vitamin C	1.3 mg
Potassium	148 mg
Beta-carotene	54 mcg
Calcium	22 mg
Magnesium	11 mg

MAJOR NUTRIENTS PER 3½ oz/100 G DRIED FIGS

Kcalories	210
Total fat	Trace
Protein	0.5 g
Carbohydrate	12.3 g
Fiber	7 g
Vitamin C	1.3 mg
Potassium	148 mg
Beta-carotene	54 mcg
Calcium	22 mg
Magnesium	11 mg

FIGS

Fresh and dried figs are rich in fiber and high in iron, boosting energy and promoting healthy blood.

Figs are usually available dried, as fresh figs are easily damaged and have a very short shelf life. This delicious fruit contains good amounts of fiber, most of it soluble, which helps protect against heart disease. Figs are also a good source of several minerals and vitamin B6, with small amounts of a range of B vitamins, folate, and several other vitamins and minerals. Dried figs are a concentrated source of potassium and are rich in calcium, magnesium, and iron. They are, however, also high in calories, so are best eaten in moderation.

- Contain sterols, which help to lower blood cholesterol.
- Good source of natural energy and sugars.
- Good source of potassium to help prevent fluid retention.
- Dried fruit is an excellent source of iron, for healthy blood, and of calcium, for bone density.

Practical tips:
Fresh figs deteriorate quickly and so should be eaten the day they are bought or picked. They are best eaten as they are but are also tasty with ham, served as an appetizer, or as part of a dessert. Some varieties of fig have edible skin while others need to be skinned.

Broiled honeyed figs with sabayon

SERVES 4

8 ripe fresh figs, halved

4 tbsp honey

leaves from 2 fresh rosemary
    sprigs, finely chopped
    (optional)

3 eggs

Method

1 Preheat the broiler to high. Arrange the figs, cut-side up, on the broiler rack. Brush with half the honey and scatter over the rosemary, if using.

2 Cook under the preheated broiler for 5–6 minutes, or until just beginning to caramelize.

3 Meanwhile, make the sabayon. Lightly whisk the eggs with the remaining honey in a large, heatproof bowl, then set over a saucepan of simmering water. Using a handheld electric whisk, beat the eggs and honey together for about 10 minutes, or until pale and thick.

4 Place 4 fig halves on 4 serving plates, add a generous spoonful of the sabayon, and serve immediately.

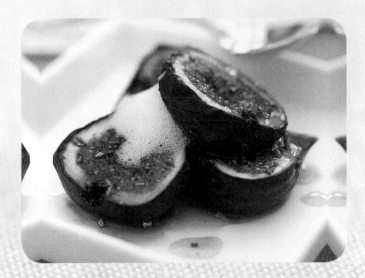

05

APRICOTS

Both fresh and dried apricots are highly nutritious and have a low glycemic index, making them an excellent food for sweet-toothed dieters.

MAJOR NUTRIENTS PER 2 AVERAGE-SIZED FRESH APRICOTS

Kcalories	31
Total fat	Trace
Protein	0.9 g
Carbohydrate	7.2 g
Fiber	1.7 g
Vitamin C	6 mg
Potassium	766 mcg
Beta-carotene	766 mcg
Iron	0.5 mg

MAJOR NUTRIENTS PER 3 SEMIDRIED APRICOTS (1¼ oz/30 G)

Kcalories	47
Total fat	Trace
Protein	1.2 g
Carbohydrate	10.8 g
Fiber	1.9 g
Vitamin C	Trace
Potassium	414 mg
Beta-carotene	163 mcg
Iron	1 mg

Fresh apricots contain vitamin C, folate, potassium, and vitamin E. Their high content of beta-carotene, an important antioxidant, helps to prevent some cancers. They are also ideal for weight maintenance as they are a good source of fiber and are fat-free. The semidried, plumped fruit is a very good source of potassium and iron, although the drying process diminishes the vitamin C and carotene content. Dried apricots, because they contain less water, are, weight for weight, higher in calories than fresh ones, but they are an ideal energy-giving snack.

- Contain a range of carotenes: beta-carotene for cancer prevention; lutein and zeaxanthin for eye health; and cryptoxanthin, which may help to maintain bone health.
- High in total and soluble fiber for healthy heart and circulation.
- Excellent source of potassium.

Practical tips:
Fresh apricots need to be fully ripe to maximize their carotene content, and cooking them helps the carotene and soluble fiber to be better absorbed in the body. Fresh apricots are excellent in fruit crumbles or poached in white wine. When buying dried apricots, ideally choose organic varieties, because these do not contain sulfur dioxide, to which some people are allergic. Dried apricots are good in couscous, salads, and can be stewed then served with yogurt.

Apricot buzz

SERVES 1–2

6 apricots

1 orange

1 fresh lemongrass stalk

¾-inch/2-cm piece fresh ginger, peeled

Method

1 Halve and pit the apricots. Peel the orange, leaving some of the white pith. Cut the lemongrass into chunks.

2 Place the apricots, orange, lemongrass, and ginger in the juicer and juice all the ingredients together. Pour the mixture into tall glasses and serve.

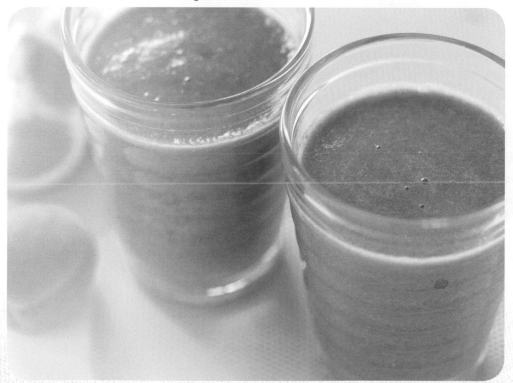

06 MANGOES

The mango is a nutritional superstar among fruits, being very rich in antioxidants and vitamins C and E.

Mangoes are grown throughout the tropics. Their orange flesh contains more antioxidant beta-carotene, which can protect against some cancers and heart disease, than most other fruits. They are high in vitamin C—one fruit can contain more than a whole day's RDA—and in fiber. Unlike most other fruits, they also contain a significant amount of the antioxidant vitamin E, which can boost the body's immune system and maintain healthy skin. Their medium–low glycemic index also means they are a good fruit for dieters as they will help regulate blood sugar levels.

- High levels of pectin—a soluble fiber that helps reduce "bad" blood cholesterol.
- Rich in potassium (320 mg per fruit) for regulating blood pressure.
- Valuable source of vitamin C.

Practical tips:
If you buy unripe mangoes, put them in a paper bag in a dark place and they will ripen within a few days. Eat ripe mangoes raw for maximum vitamin C content, or eat them with a little fat, such as whole yogurt or in a salad dressed with olive oil, to better absorb their carotenes.

DID YOU KNOW?

Mangoes contain a special enzyme that can be a soothing digestive aid—it can also help tenderize meat.

MAJOR NUTRIENTS PER AVERAGE-SIZED MANGO

Kcalories	114
Total fat	0.3 g
Protein	1.4 g
Carbohydrate	28 g
Fiber	5.2 g
Vitamin C	74 mg

Mango and tomato salsa

SERVES 4–6

6 medium ripe tomatoes

1 tbsp olive oil

1 onion, finely chopped

1 large mango, halved, seeded,
*   peeled, and diced*

2 tbsp chopped fresh cilantro

salt and pepper

tortilla chips, to serve

Method

1 Place the tomatoes in a large bowl. Cover with boiling water and let stand for 1 minute, then lift out. Using a knife, pierce the skin and peel it off. Cut the tomato into quarters, then cut out the central core and seeds. Chop the remaining flesh and place in a large bowl.

2 Heat the oil in a skillet. Add the onion and gently fry until softened. Add to the bowl of tomatoes with the mango and cilantro. Season to taste with salt and pepper. Serve cold with tortilla chips.

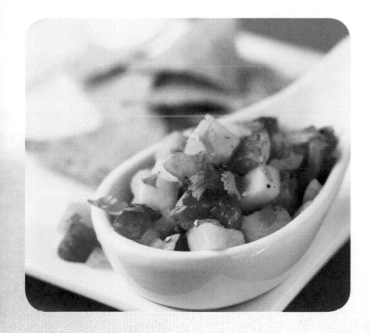

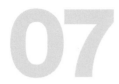

07

PEARS

This fruit—known to be hypoallergenic—is antibacterial, high in fiber, and contains antioxidants to help prevent cancer and gastroenteritis.

Pear cultivation goes back over 3,000 years in western Asia, and there has been some evidence of its discovery as far back as the Stone Age. Pears are closely related to apples and there are many varieties. It has been found that, compared to many other fruits, they are less likely to produce an adverse or allergic response from eating them, and this makes them particularly useful as a first fruit for young children. They contain a range of useful nutrients and a good amount of fiber, which helps maintain a healthy colon.

- Safe fruit for most children and for people who suffer from food allergies.
- A good source of a range of nutrients, including vitamin C and potassium.
- Contain hydroxycinnamic acids, antioxidants that are anticancer and antibacterial and may help prevent gastroenteritis.

Practical tips:
Pears don't ripen well on the tree, so bought pears tend to be under-ripe. Place them in a cool to moderately warm room and once ripe they should be eaten within a day—they tend to spoil quickly. Pears can also brown easily—to prevent this, sprinkle the cut sides with lemon juice. Although an ideal snack or lunch box fruit, pears are very versatile and can be baked, sautéed, or poached, used in mixed fruit compotes, crumbles, and pies.

DID YOU KNOW?

Much of the fiber in pears is contained in the skin, so it is best to simply wash the fruit and not peel it.

MAJOR NUTRIENTS PER AVERAGE-SIZED PEAR

Kcalories	60
Total fat	Trace
Protein	0.5 g
Carbohydrate	15 g
Fiber	3.3 g
Vitamin C	9 mg
Potassium	225 mg

Aromatic pears

SERVES 4

4 ripe but firm pears, about
*   5 oz/140 g each*
2 tbsp lemon juice
1 tbsp honey, or to taste
1 fresh red jalapeño chile, cut
*   in half and seeded*
2 whole star anise
1 cinnamon stick, bruised
1 lemongrass stalk, bruised
½-inch/1-cm piece fresh ginger,
*   peeled and sliced*
2 whole cloves
4 fresh bay leaves
1¼ cups water

Method

1 Using a vegetable peeler, peel the pears as thinly as possible and leave the stalk intact. If necessary, cut off a thin slice from the base of each pear so it will stand upright. Place in a large bowl and pour over the lemon juice with enough water to cover the pears.

2 Pour the honey into a large saucepan with a lid. Add the chile, star anise, cinnamon stick, lemongrass, ginger, cloves, bay leaves, and water. Bring to a boil, then reduce the heat and simmer, stirring occasionally, for 5 minutes, or until the honey has dissolved.

3 Drain the pears and place in the pan. Bring almost to boiling point, then reduce the heat to a gentle simmer and cover with the lid.

4 Cook for 15–20 minutes, or until the pears are tender. Remove the pan from the heat and let the pears cool in the syrup. When cool, remove them from the pan with a slotted spoon and place in a serving dish.

5 Return the syrup to the heat and bring to a boil. Boil for 5–8 minutes, or until the syrup has reduced by half and thickened. Let cool for 5–10 minutes, then pour over the pears and serve.

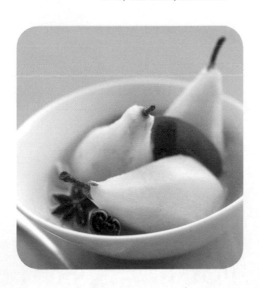

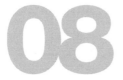

PAPAYAS

The tropical papaya, sometimes called pawpaw, is extremely high in carotenes, which are linked with cancer prevention and healthy lungs and eyes.

The papaya flesh is high in fructose (fruit sugars) and relatively high in calories, so it's good as a hunger-beating snack or dessert. The flesh is also high in carotenes, which can help prevent cancer, and it is a good source of fiber. In addition, it is one of the richest fruits in potassium and much higher in calcium than most other fruits. Papaya is also extremely high in vitamin C, and has a reasonable source of magnesium and vitamin E. It contains the enzyme papain, which breaks down protein and tenderizes meat.

- Rich in beta-carotene, which can help prevent prostate cancer.
- A good source of the carotenes lutein and zeaxanthin, which can help protect eyes from macular degeneration.
- Rich in beta-cryptoxanthin, which can help maintain healthy lungs and may help prevent arthritis.
- Excellent source of vitamin C and fiber.
- High soluble fiber content helps control blood sugar levels by slowing sugar absorption.

Practical tips:
When a papaya is ripe, its skin is orange, rather than green. It can be added to a casserole to tenderize the meat. In a fruit salad, add just before serving—the papain in it can oversoften other fruits. The papain also prevents gelatin setting, so avoid using it in gelatin desserts. Lime juice sprinkled on the fruit brings out its flavor.

DID YOU KNOW?

Papaya seeds can be dried in an oven on low heat and used like peppercorns.

MAJOR NUTRIENTS PER AVERAGE-SIZED PAPAYA

Kcalories	120
Total fat	0.4 g
Protein	1.5 g
Carbohydrate	30 g
Fiber	5.5 g
Vitamin C	180 mg
Potassium	780 mg
Beta-carotene	839 mcg
Beta-cryptoxanthin	2313 mcg
Magnesium	30 mg
Lutein/Zeaxanthin	228 mcg

Papaya and banana smoothie

SERVES 2

1 papaya
juice of 1 lime
1 large banana
1½ cups freshly squeezed
  orange juice
¼ tsp ground ginger

Method

1 Halve the papaya and scoop out and discard the gray-black seeds. Scoop out the flesh and chop coarsely, then toss with the lime juice. Peel and slice the banana.

2 Place the papaya, banana, orange juice, and ginger in a blender and process until thoroughly combined. Pour the mixture into chilled glasses and serve immediately.

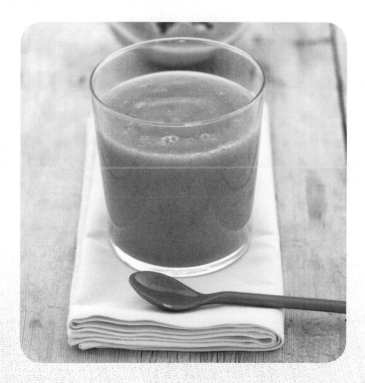

09 ORANGES

Vitamin C, the antioxidant vitamin that boosts the immune system and protects from the signs of aging, is found in abundance in oranges.

Oranges are one of the least expensive sources of vitamin C, which protects against cell damage, aging, and disease. The fruit is also a good source of fiber, folate, and potassium as well as calcium, which is vital for bone maintenance. They contain the carotenes zeaxanthin and lutein, both of which can help maintain eye health and protect against macular degeneration. Oranges also contain rutin, a flavonoid that can help slow down or prevent the growth of tumors, and nobiletin, an anti-inflammatory compound. All these plant compounds also help vitamin C to work more effectively.

- Can help prevent infections and the severity and duration of colds may be lessened by increasing intake of vitamin C.
- Oranges are one of the few fruits that are low on the glycemic index, so they are a useful food for dieters and diabetics.
- Good content of soluble fiber pectin, which helps control blood cholesterol levels.
- Anti-inflammatory, so may help reduce incidence of arthritis.
- Blood oranges contain even higher levels of antioxidants in red anthocyanin pigments, which are linked with cancer prevention.

Practical tips:
Buy oranges that feel heavy to hold compared with their size—this means they should be juicy and fresh. Store them in the refrigerator to retain their vitamin C. Orange peel contains high levels of nutrients, but should be scrubbed and dried before use.

DID YOU KNOW?

You should eat some of the white pith of the orange as well as the juicy flesh because it contains high levels of fiber, useful plant chemicals, and antioxidants.

MAJOR NUTRIENTS PER AVERAGE-SIZED ORANGE

Kcalories	65
Total fat	Trace
Protein	1 g
Carbohydrate	16 g
Fiber	3.4 g
Vitamin C	64 mg
Potassium	238 mg
Calcium	61 mg
Lutein/Zeaxanthin	182 mcg

Orange and carrot stir-fry

SERVES 4

2 tbsp peanut oil
1 lb/450 g carrots, grated
8 oz/225 g leeks, shredded
2 oranges, peeled and segmented
2 tbsp tomato ketchup
1 tbsp raw brown sugar
2 tbsp light soy sauce
½ cup peanuts, chopped

Method

1 Heat a large wok over high heat for 30 seconds. Add the oil, swirl it around to coat the bottom, and heat for 30 seconds. Add the grated carrot and leeks and stir-fry for 2–3 minutes, or until the vegetables are just soft.

2 Add the orange segments to the wok and heat through gently, ensuring that you do not break up the orange segments as you stir the mixture.

3 Mix the tomato ketchup, sugar, and soy sauce together in a small bowl. Add the tomato ketchup mixture to the wok and stir-fry for 2 minutes.

4 Transfer the stir-fry to 4 warmed serving bowls and sprinkle over the chopped peanuts. Serve immediately.

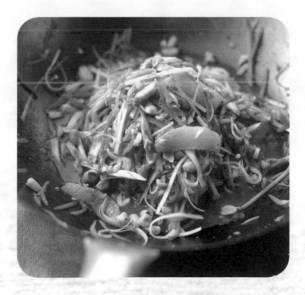

10 PINEAPPLES

A special compound found within pineapples can help ease the pain of arthritis and may help to prevent strokes.

Pineapples have long been used as a medicinal plant in various parts of the world, particularly the Americas. Apart from being a good source of vitamin C and various other vitamins and minerals, including magnesium, the pineapple contains an active substance known as bromelain. This protein has been proven to ease the inflammation associated with arthritis and joint pain, and may also help to reduce the incidence of blood clots, which can lead to heart attack and strokes. Unfortunately, the inedible stem is the richest source of bromelain, but there is also a little in the fruit.

• May aid digestion and limit pain from arthritis and joint conditions.
• Can help to reduce the risk of blood clots.
• Good source of the antioxidant vitamin C.
• Good source of ferulic acid, which can help prevent cancer.

Practical tips:
A pineapple is ripe to eat when a leaf is easily pulled from the top. To prepare, cut off the leafy top and a small layer of the base, and then slice off the tough skin and "eyes." Once cut into slices, remove the chewy central core. Avoid using fresh pineapple in gelatin—the bromelain enzyme prevents setting. Canned pineapple contains no bromelain but retains much of its vitamin C. Pineapples are delicious simply served fresh, chopped with cereal or yogurt for breakfast, or try them cooked in brown sugar and a little butter for a tasty warm dessert.

DID YOU KNOW?

The bromelain in pineapples is an effective meat tenderizer—use a few spoonfuls of juice and add to meat stews and curries.

MAJOR NUTRIENTS PER AVERAGE-SIZED PINEAPPLE SLICE

Kcalories	40
Total fat	Trace
Protein	0.5 g
Carbohydrate	10.6 g
Fiber	1.2 g
Vitamin C	30 mg
Potassium	97 mg
Magnesium	10 mg

Broiled pineapple with nutty yogurt

SERVES 4–6

1 fresh pineapple

canola oil, for brushing

⅔ cup low-fat Greek-style yogurt

¾ cup hazelnuts, skinned and
    coarsely chopped

Method

1 Cut off the leaf top from the pineapple and discard. Cut the pineapple into slices ¾ inches/2 cm thick. Using a sharp knife, cut off the skin from each slice, then, holding the slices on their sides, cut out and discard the "eyes." Stamp out the core with an apple corer or cookie cutter and cut each slice in half.

2 Brush the broiler rack with oil and preheat the broiler to high. Mix the yogurt and hazelnuts together in a bowl and set aside until needed.

3 Arrange the pineapple slices on the broiler rack and cook under the preheated broiler for 3–5 minutes, until golden. Serve with the nutty yogurt.

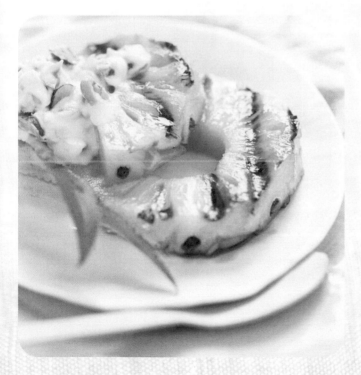

11

LEMONS

Indispensable in many recipes, lemons are rich in vitamin C and can help protect us from breast and other cancers.

The fresh, acidic flavor of lemon juice enhances both sweet and savory foods and dishes, while the peel can be used to add flavor. The acid and antioxidants in lemon juice means that it can help prevent foods from browning once peeled or cut. All parts of the lemon contain valuable nutrients and antioxidants. They are a particularly good source of vitamin C. The plant compound antioxidants include limonene, an oil that may help to prevent breast and other cancers and lower "bad" blood cholesterol, and rutin, which has been found to strengthen veins. Lemons stimulate the taste buds and may be useful for people with a poor appetite.

- Rich in vitamin C.
- Contain disinfecting and insecticide properties.
- Rutin content may help to strengthen veins and prevent fluid retention, especially in the legs.
- Help increase appetite.

Practical tips:
Either wash thoroughly or buy unwaxed or organic lemons if you want to use the peel. You can get more juice from a lemon if you warm it for a few seconds, in the microwave or in hot water, before squeezing. The heavier the lemon, the more juice it should contain. Lemon juice, thanks to its pectin, helps jams and jellies to set, can be used instead of vinegar in salad dressings, or added to mayonnaise.

DID YOU KNOW?

An average lemon contains about 3 tablespoons of juice. The tenderizing acid in lemons makes a useful addition to marinades for meat, or meat stews.

MAJOR NUTRIENTS PER AVERAGE-SIZED LEMON

Kcalories	17
Total fat	Trace
Protein	0.6 g
Carbohydrate	5.4 g
Fiber	1.6 g
Vitamin C	31 mg
Potassium	80 mg

Lemon and orange peppered monkfish

SERVES 8 (D) (P) (C)

2 lemons
2 oranges
2 monkfish tails, about
    1 lb 2 oz/500 g each,
    skinned and cut into
    4 fillets
8 fresh lemon thyme sprigs
2 tbsp olive oil
2 tbsp green peppercorns,
    lightly crushed
salt

Method

1 Cut 8 lemon slices and 8 orange slices, reserving the remaining fruit. Rinse the monkfish fillets under cold running water and pat dry with paper towels. Place the monkfish fillets, cut-side up, on a work surface and divide the citrus slices among them. Top with the lemon thyme. Tie each fillet at intervals with kitchen string to secure the citrus slices and thyme. Place the monkfish in a large, shallow, nonmetallic dish.

2 Squeeze the juice from the remaining fruit into a pitcher, add the oil, and mix together. Season to taste with salt, then spoon the mixture over the fish. Cover with plastic wrap and let marinate in the refrigerator for up to 1 hour, spooning the marinade over the fish tails once or twice.

3 Preheat the broiler. Drain the fish, reserving the marinade. Sprinkle the crushed peppercorns over the fish, pressing them in with your fingers, then cook over medium–high heat, turning and brushing frequently with the marinade, for 20–25 minutes. Transfer to a cutting board, remove and discard the string, and cut the fish into slices. Serve immediately.

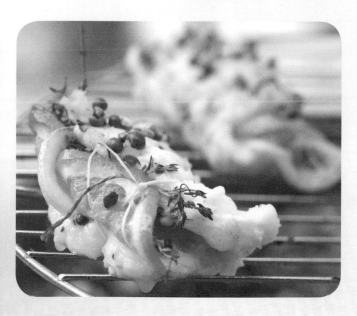

12 GRAPEFRUITS

An excellent source of vitamin C, eating grapefruit boosts the immune system and protects our hearts.

In recent years, the pink-fleshed grapefruit has become as popular as the white or yellow-fleshed variety. It is a little sweeter and contains more health benefits—the pink pigment indicates the presence of lycopene, the antioxidant carotene that has been shown to help prevent prostate and other cancers. Like other citrus fruits, grapefruits contain bioflavonoids, compounds that appear to increase the benefits of vitamin C, also found in this fruit in excellent amounts. Grapefruits are low on the glycemic index and very low in calories, so make an important fruit for dieters. Because grapefruit juice can alter the effect of certain drugs (e.g. drugs that lower blood pressure), people on medication should check with their doctors before they consume the fruit.

- High in antioxidants, which can help prevent prostate and other cancers.
- Rich in vitamin C to boost the immune system.
- Excellent fruit for dieters.
- Help reduce bouts of wheezing in asthma-prone people.

Practical tips:
Grapefruit is delicious halved, sprinkled with dark brown sugar and broiled for a short while. Try to eat some of the white pith with your grapefruit because this is high in nutrients. Grapefruits, like all citrus fruits, will contain more juice if they feel heavier.

DID YOU KNOW?

The slightly bitter taste of some grapefruits is caused by a compound called naringenin, which has cholesterol-lowering properties.

MAJOR NUTRIENTS PER HALF PINK GRAPEFRUIT

Kcalories	30
Total fat	Trace
Protein	0.5 g
Carbohydrate	7.5 g
Fiber	1.1 g
Vitamin C	37 mg
Potassium	127 mg
Beta-carotene	770 mcg
Folate	9 mcg
Calcium	15 mg

Grapefruit and orange salad

SERVES 4

1 pink grapefruit
1 yellow grapefruit
3 oranges

Method

1 Using a sharp knife, carefully cut away all the peel and pith from the grapefruits and oranges.

2 Working over a bowl to catch the juice, carefully cut the grapefruit and orange segments between the membranes to obtain skinless segments of fruit. Discard any seeds. Add the segments to the bowl and gently mix together. Cover and let chill in the refrigerator until required or divide among 4 serving dishes and serve.

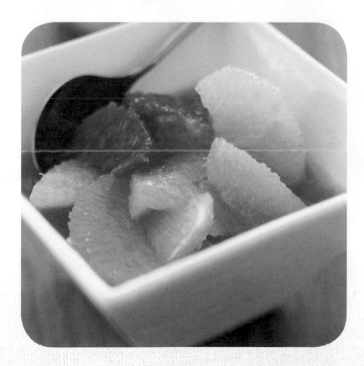

13 CHERRIES

Glossy red cherries are one of the best fruit sources of antioxidants, which help prevent many diseases associated with aging.

Although cherries contain slightly smaller amounts of vitamins and minerals than other pit fruits, they are rich in several plant compounds that have definite health benefits. They rank highly— in twelfth place—on the ORAC scale of antioxidant capacity in fruits, and the chemicals they contain include quercetin: a flavonoid that has anticancer and heart-protecting qualities; and cyanidin, which is an anti-inflammatory that minimizes symptoms of arthritis and gout. The soluble fiber contained in cherries is helpful for controlling "bad" blood cholesterol levels, while the fruit is also a good source of potassium and a reasonable source of vitamin C and carotenes.

- High in antioxidants, which help protect the heart and prevent signs of aging.
- Rich in quercetin to help prevent cancers.
- Rich in cyanidin to alleviate arthritis and inflammatory diseases.
- Soluble fiber helps improve blood cholesterol profile.

Practical tips:
Fresh cherries will have green stalks and a glossy skin. The deeper the color, the more antioxidant compounds they contain, so choose red or black, rather than yellow, cherries. To preserve vitamin C, store in the refrigerator. Fresh cherries contain higher levels of antioxidants, so are best eaten raw.

DID YOU KNOW?

Morello cherries are a sour, rather than sweet, variety of cherry and are usually used in pies and cooking.

MAJOR NUTRIENTS PER 3 oz/80 G CHERRIES

Kcalories	50
Total fat	Trace
Protein	0.8 g
Carbohydrate	13 g
Fiber	1.7 g
Vitamin C	5.6 mg
Potassium	178 mg
Lutein/Zeaxanthin	68 mcg

Cherry pink

SERVES 1–2

3 cups dark sweet cherries
½ lime
1 apple
½ heaping cup red grapes
2½ heaping tbsp soy yogurt

Method

1 Pit the cherries. Halve the lime. Juice the apple, cherries, grapes, and lime together. Whisk in the yogurt, pour the mixture into glasses, and serve.

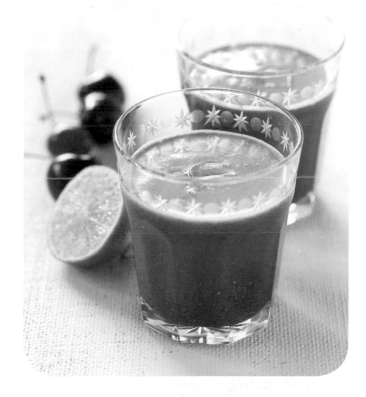

14 STRAWBERRIES

Rich in vitamin C, strawberries boost the immune system and contain chemicals that offer cancer protection.

Strawberries rank very high in antioxidant activity. They are extremely rich in vitamin C (an average portion contains the entire recommended daily amount for an adult) and this helps to boost the immune system and help wound healing, prevent arterial damage, promote iron absorption, and strengthen blood vessel walls. They also contain other antioxidant phenolic plant chemicals such as anthocyanins and ellagic acid, which can block cancer cells and help prevent some cancers. Lastly, they contain good amounts of fiber, folate, and potassium.

DID YOU KNOW?

Once washed, strawberries will spoil quickly—only wash immediately before serving.

- Excellent source of vitamin C.
- Contain ellagic acid, a compound with anticancer and antioxidant properties.
- Contain anthocyanins, which can help lower "bad" blood cholesterol.
- Useful source of fiber and soluble fiber, potassium, folate, and zeaxanthin for healthy eyes.

Practical tips:

Choose strawberries that look plump and glossy; dull ones are usually past their best. Smaller strawberries tend to have higher levels of ellagic acid, concentrated in the outer layer, and have more flavor. Store in a container with air holes, in a refrigerator, for up to three days, but bring them to room temperature before using.

MAJOR NUTRIENTS PER 3½ oz/100 G STRAWBERRIES

Kcalories	32
Total fat	0.3
Protein	0.7 g
Carbohydrate	7.7 g
Fiber	2 g
Vitamin C	59 mg
Potassium	153 mg
Folate	24 mcg
Lutein/Zeaxanthin	26 mcg

Strawberry and balsamic vinegar semifreddo

SERVES 4

1 tsp honey
⅓ cup water
scant 3¼ cups ripe
  strawberries, hulled
2 tbsp balsamic vinegar
4 strawberries, halved, and
  fresh mint sprigs, to decorate
  (optional)

Method

1 Set the freezer to rapid freeze at least 2 hours before freezing. Pour the honey and water into a saucepan and bring to a boil, stirring occasionally. Reduce the heat to a simmer, then add the strawberries and simmer for 2 minutes. Remove from the heat and let cool.

2 Place the strawberries and syrup in a food processor with the balsamic vinegar and process for 30 seconds, or until a chunky mixture is formed.

3 Pour the mixture into a freezerproof container and freeze for 1–1½ hours, or until semifrozen. Stir at least once during freezing.

4 Scoop spoonfuls of the semifreddo into glasses, decorate with halved strawberries and mint sprigs, if using, and serve. Remember to return the freezer to its original setting.

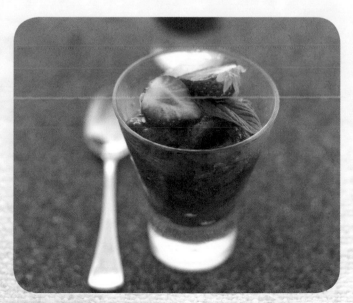

15 RASPBERRIES

Packed with vitamin C, fiber, and antioxidants to protect the heart, raspberries are one of the most nutritious fruits.

Raspberries are the seventh-highest fruit on the ORAC scale. They are therefore an extremely covetable fruit and best eaten raw, because cooking or processing destroys some of these antioxidants, especially anthocyanins. Anthocyanins are red and purple pigments that have been shown to help prevent both heart disease and cancers, and may also help prevent varicose veins. Raspberries also contain high levels of ellagic acid, a compound with anticancer properties. In addition, they are high in vitamin C and fiber, and contain good amounts of iron, which the body absorbs well because of the high levels of vitamin C.

- High antioxidant activity.
- May help to prevent varicose veins.
- One portion contains approximately half a day's recommended intake of vitamin C.
- High in fiber to help control high "bad" cholesterol.

Practical tips:
The berries do not keep for long, so should only be picked when ripe. They do freeze very well though, if packed in containers rather than plastic bags. Never wash raspberries before storing unless absolutely necessary—their structure is easily destroyed. The healthy soluble fiber in raspberries is pectin, which means they make excellent, easy-to-set jam.

DID YOU KNOW?

Raspberries consist of numerous smaller fruits called drupelets, which are clustered around a central stalk core. Each drupelet contains a seed, which is why raspberries are so high in fiber.

MAJOR NUTRIENTS PER 3½ oz/100 G RASPBERRIES

Kcalories	52
Total fat	0.6 g
Protein	1.2 g
Carbohydrate	12 g
Fiber	6.5 g
Vitamin C	26 mg
Vitamin B3	0.6 mg
Vitamin E	0.8 mg
Folate	21 mcg
Potassium	151 mg
Calcium	25 mg
Iron	0.7 mg
Zinc	0.4 mg

Raspberry and pear delight

SERVES 2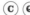

2 large ripe Anjou or Bartlett pears
½ cup frozen raspberries
generous ⅓ cup ice-cold water
honey, to taste (optional)
fresh raspberries, for decorating
(optional)

Method

1 Peel and quarter the pears, removing the cores. Place the pears in a blender with the raspberries and water and process until smooth.

2 Taste and sweeten with honey if the raspberries are a little sharp. Pour into chilled glasses, decorate with raspberries, if using, and serve.

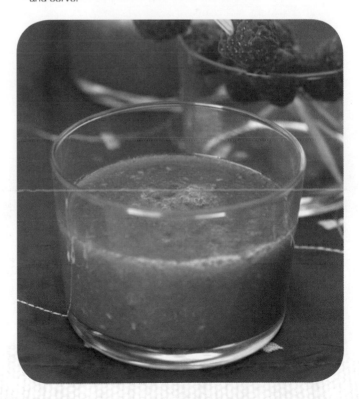

16

BLUEBERRIES

These deep purple berries are the richest of all fruits in antioxidant compounds, which protect us from cancers and several other diseases.

The wild blueberry has become one of the most popular berries. They are the third-highest plant food on the ORAC scale so just a handful of berries a day can offer protection from some diseases. The compound pterostilbene, which is found in the fruit, could be as effective as commercial drugs in lowering cholesterol, and may also help prevent diabetes and some cancers. Blueberries are a good source of anthocyanins, which can help prevent heart disease and memory loss. They are high in vitamin C and fiber and also appear to help urinary tract infections.

- Contain a cholesterol-lowering compound.
- Can help prevent coronary heart disease, diabetes, and cancers.
- Help beat urinary tract infections.
- Appear to help protect against intestinal upsets, including food poisoning.
- Their carotene, in the form of lutein and zeaxanthin, helps keep eyes healthy.

Practical tips:
Blueberries are quite sweet so can be eaten raw, which helps to preserve their vitamin C content. They can also be lightly cooked in a small amount of water and eaten with the juices. Blueberries can boost the nutrient content of muffins, cakes, crumbles, pies, and fruit salads. The berries freeze well and lose few of their nutrients.

DID YOU KNOW?

Blueberries should be stored in a nonmetallic container—contact with metal can discolor them.

MAJOR NUTRIENTS PER 1¾ oz/50 G BLUEBERRIES

Kcalories	29
Total fat	Trace
Protein	0.4 g
Carbohydrate	7.2 g
Fiber	1.2 g
Vitamin C	5 mg
Vitamin E	2.4 mg
Folate	34 mcg
Potassium	39 mg
Lutein/Zeaxanthin	40 mcg

Yogurt with blueberries, honey, and nuts

SERVES 4

3 tbsp honey
½ cup mixed unsalted nuts
8 tbsp low-fat Greek-style yogurt
heaping 1⅓ cups fresh blueberries

Method

1 Heat the honey in a small saucepan over medium heat. Add the nuts and stir until they are well coated. Remove from the heat and let cool slightly.

2 Divide the yogurt among 4 serving bowls, then spoon over the nut mixture and the blueberries.

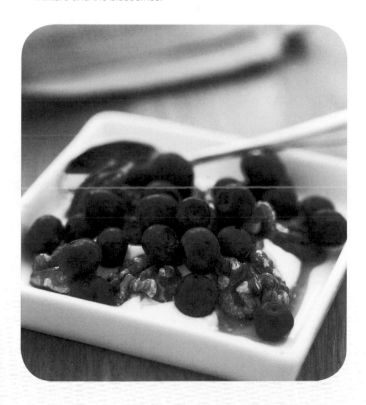

17

CRANBERRIES

These small red fruits have a variety of health benefits and help to boost the work of the kidneys.

DID YOU KNOW?

People taking warfarin should avoid eating cranberries or drinking cranberry juice—the berry can raise blood levels of this anticoagulant drug to a very high, possibly fatal, degree.

MAJOR NUTRIENTS IN GENEROUS ¾ CUP SWEETENED CRANBERRY JUICE

Kcalories	108
Total fat	Trace
Protein	Trace
Carbohydrate	26 g
Fiber	Trace
Vitamin C	60 mg
Vitamin E	Trace
Lutein/Zeaxanthin	150 mcg

PER 3½ oz/100 G RAW CRANBERRIES

Kcalories	46
Total fat	Trace
Protein	0.4 g
Carbohydrate	12.2 g
Fiber	4.6 g
Vitamin C	13 mg
Vitamin E	1.2 mg
Lutein/Zeaxanthin	91 mcg

Fresh cranberries are too sour and acidic to eat as they are but, for many years, they have been used as a sauce to serve with turkey. However, since their health-giving properties were discovered, they are now widely found sweetened and dried, as a juice drink, and in baked desserts and preserves. Their best-known benefit is that they can help to prevent, or alleviate, urinary tract infections. This is partly because they contain quinic acid, which increases the acidity of the urine, and partly because of the tannins they contain, which are antibacterial. The same compounds may also help protect against stomach ulcers and heart disease.

• High soluble fiber content may help reduce "bad" cholesterol.
• May protect against heart disease.
• Help prevent and alleviate urinary tract infections.
• Help prevent digestive disorders and stomach ulcers.

Practical tips:
Cranberries sold fresh should have a smooth, bright skin. It is said that one way to test their freshness is to drop one—if it bounces, it is fresh! Cranberries are rich in pectin, and make a valuable addition to jams made with low-pectin fruit, such as strawberries, to help them set. The sugar content of most cranberry products, such as drinks and dried fruit, is relatively high in calories and may not be suitable for people on a low-calorie or low sugar diet.

Cranberry booster

SERVES 2

3¾ cups cranberries,
    thawed if frozen
generous 1¾ cups unsweetened
    cranberry juice, chilled
1¼ cups plain yogurt
2–3 tbsp honey, or to taste

Method

1 Place the berries and juice in a blender and process until smooth. Add the yogurt and honey and process again until combined.

2 Taste and add more honey, if necessary. Pour the mixture into chilled glasses and serve immediately.

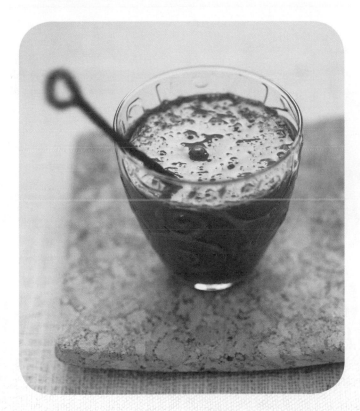

18 PLUMS

Research shows that antioxidents found in plums protect the brain as well as the heart.

Plums come in a variety of colors, from the more common red and purple varieties to yellow and white. The fruits are well known for their health-giving phenolic compounds—neochlorogenic and chlorogenic acids—which are particularly effective in neutralizing free radicals, which contribute to disease and the aging process. They seem to be especially beneficial in their antioxidant action on the fatty tissues in the brain and help prevent damage to fats circulating in our blood. The red and purple varieties are also rich in anthocyanins, the pigments that help to prevent heart disease and cancers.

- Low glycemic index is useful for dieters and diabetics.
- Good source of carotenes for cancer protection and eye health.
- Rich in phenolic compounds for healthy brain and strong antioxidant action.
- Source of easily absorbed iron for healthy blood and body maintenance.

Practical tips:
Buy plums that are almost ripe, preferably still with a slight bloom on the skin, and allow to ripen at room temperature for one to two days—fully ripe plums contain the most antioxidants. Plums bought for cooking should be poached in a little water and eaten with the juices because some of the nutrients will leach into the water.

DID YOU KNOW?

Plums, native to China and Europe, have been eaten for at least 2,000 years. There are also over 2,000 varieties.

MAJOR NUTRIENTS PER AVERAGE-SIZED PLUM

Kcalories	30
Total fat	Trace
Protein	0.5 g
Carbohydrate	7.5 g
Fiber	0.9 g
Vitamin C	6.3 mg
Beta-carotene	125 mcg
Potassium	104 mg
Iron	0.4 mcg
Zeaxanthin/Lutein	48 mcg

Dark plum compote

SERVES 4

1 lb 5 oz/600 g dark-skinned
plums, halved and pitted
lightly low-fat whipped cream
or sour cream, to serve

Syrup
¾ cup sugar
1¾ cups water
3 fresh bay leaves, torn
1 thinly pared strip of orange zest

Method

1 Place the plum halves in a large serving bowl.

2 Heat the syrup ingredients together in a saucepan over medium heat, stirring, until the sugar has dissolved. Bring to a boil and boil for 7–10 minutes, or until syrupy. Immediately strain the boiling syrup over the plums and let cool to room temperature. Serve with lightly whipped cream.

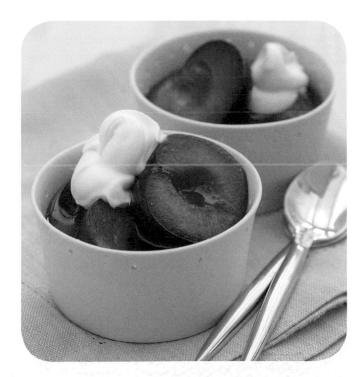

19

MELONS

The juicy flesh of the melon is rich in vitamin C and is a great source of potassium to help prevent fluid retention.

A melon contains over 92 percent water, which can help keep the kidneys working well. The orange varieties are a great source of beta-carotene and are also high in vitamin C, although amounts vary according to variety. All melons are rich in vitamin B6 and potassium and several varieties are high in the bioflavonoid group of plant chemicals, which have anticancer, anti-heart disease, and anti-aging properties. Melons are also rich in soluble fiber, while watermelon is a particularly good source of lycopene, which helps protect against prostate cancer.

- High potassium content helps prevent fluid retention and balances sodium in the body.
- Soluble fiber content helps arterial health and can help lower "bad" blood cholesterol.
- Beta-carotene content of orange varieties is one of the highest of all fruits and vegetables.
- Watermelon contains citrulline, an amino acid that aids blood flow to muscles, helpful for exercise and sports.

Practical tips:
Unlike many fruits, melons don't ripen once picked, so choose one with a rich fragrance, which indicates it is ripe. If it has wrinkles, it is overripe. Store melons at cool to moderate room temperature.

DID YOU KNOW?
If you buy half or a quarter of a melon, it should be stored well wrapped in plastic wrap in the refrigerator to prevent other foods from absorbing its strong odor.

MAJOR NUTRIENTS PER AVERAGE-SIZED CANTALOUPE MELON

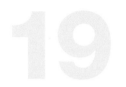

Kcalories	28
Total fat	Trace
Protein	1 g
Carbohydrate	6.3 g
Fiber	1.5 g
Vitamin C	39 mg
Potassium	315 mg
Beta-carotene	2647 mcg

Prosciutto ham with melon and asparagus

SERVES 4

8 oz/225 g asparagus spears

1 small or ½ medium
    cantaloupe melon

2 oz/55 g Prosciutto ham,
    thinly sliced

5½ oz/150 g bag mixed
    salad greens, such as herb
    salad with arugula

¾ cup fresh raspberries

1 tbsp freshly shaved Parmesan
    cheese

Dressing

1 tbsp balsamic vinegar

2 tbsp raspberry vinegar

2 tbsp orange juice

Method

1　Trim the asparagus, cutting the spears in half if very long. Cook in a tall saucepan of lightly salted, boiling water over medium heat for 5 minutes, or until tender. Drain, then refresh under cold running water and drain again. Set aside.

2　Cut the melon in half and scoop out the seeds. Cut into small wedges and cut away the rind. Separate the Prosciutto ham slices, cut in half, and wrap around the melon wedges.

3　Arrange the salad greens on a large serving platter and place the melon wedges on top, together with the asparagus spears. Sprinkle over the raspberries and Parmesan shavings.

4　To make the dressing, pour the vinegars and juice into a screw-top jar and shake until blended. Pour over the salad and serve.

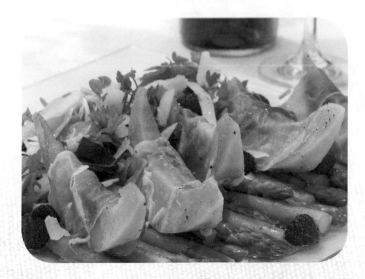

20 BLACKBERRIES

Juicy blackberries are small powerhouses of health that are rich in antioxidants to protect us from cardiovascular diseases.

In recent years it has been discovered that these tasty fruits are potent health-protectors as well as a delicious treat on a summer day. They rate almost as high on the ORAC as blueberries. Their deep purple color denotes that they are rich in several compounds, which can help beat heart disease, cancers, and the signs of aging. These compounds include anthocyanins and ellagic acid. Additionally, blackberries are rich in fiber and minerals, including magnesium, zinc, iron, and calcium. Their high vitamin E content helps protect the heart and keeps skin healthy.

• High in ellagic acid, a chemical known to block cancer cells.
• Rich in antioxidant vitamin E and fiber.
• A good source of vitamin C, which boosts the immune system.
• A useful source of folate for healthy blood.

Practical tips:
The freshest blackberries have a shiny, plump appearance. If they look dull they are likely to be past their best and the vitamin C content will be lower. The darker the blackberry, the more ellagic acid it is likely to contain. Cooking doesn't destroy ellagic acid, so you can use blackberries to make jam or in pies and crumbles. However, for maximum vitamin C they are best eaten raw. Blackberries freeze well so pack them into lidded containers or open-freeze on a tray and then pack into plastic bags.

DID YOU KNOW?

Blackberries contain salicylate, which is related to the active ingredient in aspirin. For this reason, people who are allergic to aspirin may also have a reaction to blackberries.

MAJOR NUTRIENTS PER 3½ oz/100 G BLACKBERRIES

Kcalories	25
Total fat	Trace
Protein	0.9 g
Carbohydrate	5 g
Fiber	3.1 g
Vitamin C	15 mg
Vitamin E	2.4 mg
Folate	34 mcg
Potassium	160 mg
Calcium	41 mg
Iron	0.7 mg

Very berry dessert

SERVES 6–8

*1 x ½-oz/12-g package strawberry-
flavored gelatin*
*generous ¾ cup unsweetened
cranberry juice*
*1 lb 2 oz/500 g raspberries,
strawberries, blueberries, and
blackberries, plus extra for
decorating*

Method

1 Make up the gelatin according to the package directions, but use the cranberry juice to replace some of the water. Place a mixture of berries in the bottom of individual serving glasses or plastic cups and pour over the gelatin. Let chill in the refrigerator for 6 hours until firmly set. Serve decorated with more berries.

2 To make a striped layer dessert, use 2 contrasting colored gelatins. Place one-quarter of the berries in a bowl and top with half of one gelatin. Chill until just set, then add more berries and half of the contrasting gelatin. Chill as before. Repeat twice more with the remaining gelatin, alternating the colors. Chill until firmly set.

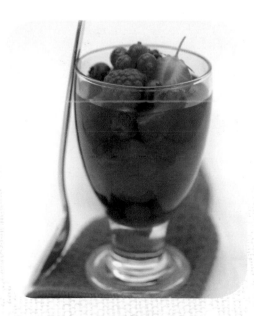

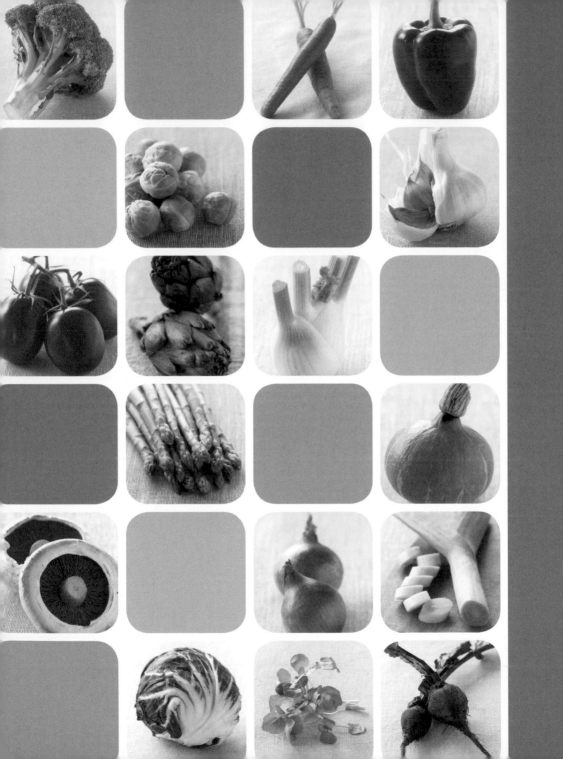

VEGETABLES AND SALADS

Carotenes, calcium, and iron are just a few of the essential health-giving properties found in vegetables and salads. Serve a portion of your favorites alongside a main dish or try any of the delicious recipes featured in this chapter.

(V) Suitable for vegetarians
(D) Ideal for dieters
(P) Suitable for pregnancy
(C) Suitable for children over 5 years
(Q) Quick to prepare and cook

21 BROCCOLI

Of all the vegetables in the brassica family, broccoli has shown the highest levels of protection against prostate cancer.

Broccoli comes in several varieties but the darker the color, the more beneficial nutrients the vegetable contains. It contains sulphoraphane and indoles, which have strong anticancer effects, particularly against breast and colon cancer. Broccoli is also high in flavonoids, which have been linked with a significant reduction in ovarian cancer. The chemicals in broccoli protect against stomach ulcers, stomach and lung cancer, and possibly skin cancer. They also act as a detoxifier, helping lower "bad" blood cholesterol, boosting the immune system, and protecting against cataracts.

- Rich in a variety of nutrients that protect against types of cancer.
- Contains chemicals that help to lower "bad" cholesterol and protect against heart disease.
- Lutein and zeaxanthin help prevent macular degeneration.
- Helps eradicate the *H.pylori* bacteria.
- High calcium content helps build and protect bones.
- Excellent source of the antioxidants vitamin C and selenium.
- 3–5 servings a week offer protection against cancer.

Practical tips:
Look for heads rich with color and avoid any broccoli with pale, yellow or brown patches on the florets. Store in the refrigerator and use within a few days of purchase. Frozen broccoli contains all the nutrients of fresh broccoli. Cook by lightly steaming or stir-frying.

DID YOU KNOW?
You can eat the leaves of the broccoli as well as the stalks and florets. They contain as much goodness and taste great, too!

MAJOR NUTRIENTS PER 3½ oz/100 G BROCCOLI

Kcalories	34
Total fat	0.4 g
Protein	2.8 g
Carbohydrate	6.6 g
Fiber	2.6 g
Vitamin C	89 mg
Selenium	2.5 mcg
Beta-carotene	361 mcg
Calcium	47 mg
Lutein/Zeaxanthin	1403 mcg

Broccoli and peanut stir-fry

SERVES 4

3 tbsp canola oil

*1 lemongrass stalk, coarsely
   chopped*

*2 fresh red chiles, seeded and
   chopped*

*1-inch/2.5-cm piece fresh ginger,
   peeled and grated*

3 kaffir lime leaves, coarsely torn

3 tbsp Thai green curry paste

1 onion, chopped

*1 red bell pepper, seeded and
   chopped*

*12 oz/350 g broccoli, cut into
   florets*

4 oz/115 g fine green beans

*heaping ⅓ cup toasted
   unsalted peanuts*

Method

1 Place 2 tablespoons of the oil, the lemongrass, chiles, ginger, lime leaves, and curry paste in a food processor or blender and process until a paste forms.

2 Heat a wok over high heat for 30 seconds. Add the remaining oil, swirl it around to coat the bottom, and heat for 30 seconds. Add the spice paste, onion, and red bell pepper and stir-fry for 2–3 minutes, until the vegetables start to soften. Add the broccoli and beans, cover, and cook over low heat for 4–5 minutes, until tender.

3 Add the peanuts to the broccoli, toss together, and serve.

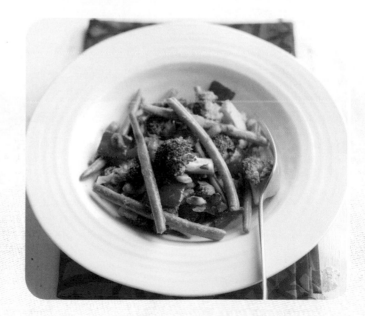

22 CARROTS

The richest in carotenes of all plant foods, carrots offer protection from cancers and cardiovascular disease, and help keep eyes and lungs healthy.

Carrots are one of the most nutritious root vegetables. They are an excellent source of antioxidant compounds, and the richest vegetable source of carotenes, which give them their bright orange color. These compounds help protect against cardiovascular disease and cancer. Carotenes may reduce the incidence of heart disease by about 45 percent, promote good vision, and help maintain healthy lungs. They are also rich in fiber, antioxidant vitamins C and E, calcium, and potassium. A chemical in carrots, falcarinol, has been shown to suppress tumors in animals by a third.

- High carotene content protects against high blood cholesterol and heart disease.
- May offer protection against some cancers and emphysema.
- Women who eat at least five carrots a week are nearly two-thirds less likely to have a stroke than those who don't.
- Carrots help to protect sight and night vision.
- Carrots contain a good range of vitamins, minerals, and fiber.

Practical tips:
The darker orange the carrot, the more carotenes it will contain. Remove any green on the stalk end of the carrot before cooking as this can be mildly toxic. The nutrients in carrots are more available to the body when a carrot is cooked, rather than raw, and adding a little oil during cooking helps the carotenes to be absorbed.

....

DID YOU KNOW?

A very high intake of carrots can cause the skin to appear orange. Called carotanemia, it is a harmless condition.

....

MAJOR NUTRIENTS PER 3½ oz/100 G CARROTS

Kcalories	41
Total fat	Trace
Protein	0.9 g
Carbohydrate	9.6 g
Fiber	2.8 g
Vitamin C	6 mg
Vitamin E	0.7 mg
Beta-carotene	8285 mcg
Calcium	33 mg
Potassium	320 mg
Lutein/Zeaxanthin	256 mcg

Gujarat carrot salad

SERVES 4–6

1 lb/450 g carrots, peeled
1 tbsp canola oil
½ tbsp black mustard seeds
½ tbsp cumin seeds
1 fresh green chile, seeded
   and chopped
½ tsp sugar
½ tsp salt
pinch of ground turmeric
1½–2 tbsp lemon juice

Method

1 Grate the carrots on the coarse side of a grater into a bowl and
set aside.

2 Heat a wok over medium–high heat for 30 seconds. Add the oil,
swirl it around to coat the bottom, and heat for 30 seconds. Add the
mustard and cumin seeds and stir-fry until the mustard seeds start
popping. Immediately remove the wok from the heat and stir in the
chile, sugar, salt, and turmeric. Let cool for 5 minutes.

3 Pour the warm spices and any oil over the carrots and add the
lemon juice. Toss together and adjust the seasoning, if necessary,
then cover and chill in the refrigerator for at least 30 minutes. Give
the salad a good toss just before serving.

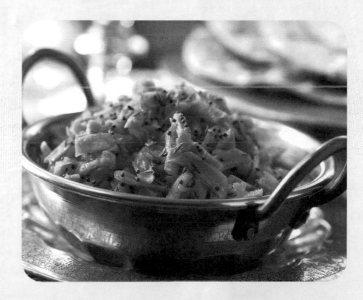

23 BELL PEPPERS

The bright colors of bell peppers contain high levels of carotenes for heart health and cancer protection, and are also a rich source of vitamin C.

Bell peppers come in a variety of colors, but red and orange bell peppers contain the highest levels of vitamin B6 and carotenes. However, all of them are extremely rich in vitamin C, with an average serving providing more than a day's recommended intake. In general, the deeper the color of the bell pepper, the more beneficial plant compounds it contains. These include bioflavonoids, to protect against cancer, and phenols, which help block the action of cancer-causing chemicals in the body. Peppers also contain plant sterols, which may have an anticancer effect.

- Rich source of a range of vitamins, minerals, and plant chemicals.
- Extremely rich in antioxidant vitamin C and excellent source of antioxidant vitamin E.
- Several components are strongly anticancer.
- High lutein levels protect from macular degeneration.
- Good source of vitamin B6 for reducing blood homocysteine levels; high levels of this have been linked to increased risk of heart disease, stroke, Alzheimer's disease, and osteoporosis.

Practical tips:
The carotenes in bell peppers are made more available to the body if peppers are cooked and eaten with a little oil. Try stir-frying thinly sliced bell peppers or seed, halve, brush with oil, and roast. If raw in a salad, drizzle over some olive oil to help absorption. Fresh bell peppers can be seeded, sliced, and frozen in plastic bags.

DID YOU KNOW?

Bell peppers are native to South America and date back about 5,000 years. They were introduced to Europe in the Middle Ages by Spanish and Portuguese explorers.

MAJOR NUTRIENTS PER AVERAGE-SIZED BELL PEPPER

Kcalories	39
Total fat	0.5 g
Protein	1.5 g
Carbohydrate	9 g
Fiber	3 g
Vitamin C	285 mg
Folate	0.7 mcg
Niacin	1.5 mg
Vitamin B6	0.44 mg
Vitamin E	2.4 mg
Potassium	317 mcg
Iron	0.7 mg
Beta-carotene	2436 mcg
Beta-cryptoxanthin	735 mcg
Lutein/Zeaxanthin	77 mcg

Red bell pepper booster

SERVES 2

generous 1 cup carrot juice
generous 1 cup tomato juice
2 large red bell peppers, seeded
    and coarsely chopped
1 tbsp lemon juice
pepper

Method

1 Pour the carrot juice and tomato juice into a food processor
  or blender and process gently until combined.

2 Add the red bell peppers and lemon juice. Season with plenty
  of pepper and process until smooth. Pour the mixture into tall
  glasses and serve.

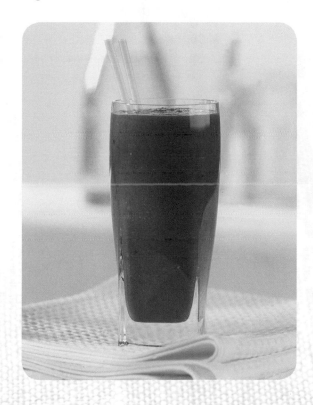

24

BRUSSELS SPROUTS

Containing many health-giving nutrients, Brussels sprouts offer high protection levels against cancers.

Brussels sprouts are an important winter vegetable, providing high levels of vitamin C and many other immune-boosting nutrients. They are rich in the sulphoraphane compound, which is a detoxifier and has been shown to help the body clear itself from potential carcinogens. Brussels sprouts have been shown to help prevent DNA damage when eaten regularly and may help minimize the spread of breast cancer. They even contain small amounts of beneficial omega-3 fats, zinc, and selenium, a mineral many adults do not eat in the recommended daily amount. People who eat large quantities of Brussels sprouts and other brassicas have a much lower risk of prostate, colorectal, and lung cancer.

- Rich in indoles and other compounds to protect against cancer; may reduce the spread of cancer.
- Extremely rich in immune-boosting vitamin C.
- Indole content can help lower "bad" blood cholesterol.
- Very high in fiber for colon health.

Practical tips:
Select bright green sprouts with tight heads and no sign of yellow leaves. Lightly steaming or quickly boiling Brussels sprouts is the best way to cook them and preserve their nutrients. Don't overcook because much of the vitamin C content will be destroyed. Overcooking also alters their flavor and gives them an unwelcome odor.

DID YOU KNOW?

Brussels sprouts are thought to come from a region in Belgium near Brussels. They were not widely used until the early 20th century.

MAJOR NUTRIENTS PER 3½ oz/100 G BRUSSELS SPROUTS

Kcalories	43
Total fat	0.3 g
Protein	3.4 g
Carbohydrate	9 g
Fiber	3.8 g
Vitamin C	85 mg
Folate	61 mcg
Magnesium	23 mg
Calcium	42 mg
Selenium	1.6 mcg
Zinc	0.4 mg
Beta-carotene	450 mcg
Lutein/Zeaxanthin	1590 mcg

Brussels sprouts with chestnuts

SERVES 4

12 oz/350 g Brussels sprouts,
*   trimmed*
2 level tbsp low-fat margarine
3½ oz/100 g canned whole
*   chestnuts, well drained or*
*   3½ oz/100 g vacuum-packed*
*   cooked chestnuts*
pinch of grated nutmeg
salt and pepper
½ cup slivered almonds,
*   to garnish*

Method

1 Cook the Brussels sprouts in a large saucepan of lightly salted, boiling water for 5 minutes. Drain thoroughly.

2 Melt the margarine in a large saucepan over medium heat. Add the Brussels sprouts and stir-fry for 3 minutes, then add the chestnuts and nutmeg. Season with salt and pepper to taste and stir well. Cook for an additional 2 minutes, then remove from the heat. Transfer to a warmed dish, scatter over the almonds, and serve.

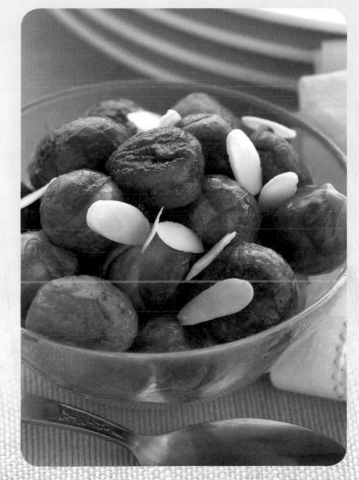

25

FAVA BEANS

The star quality of fava beans is that they are exceptionally high in fiber and can help reduce "bad" cholesterol.

Fava beans are usually podded and eaten fresh or frozen, but they can also be dried and used in a similar way to beans. Small immature pods can be cooked and eaten whole. The podded beans are very high in a form of soluble fiber called arabinose, which can help improve the blood lipid profile. They also contain the flavonoid quercetin, which can help prevent heart disease, and the beans are a good source of cancer-blocking beta-carotene, niacin (vitamin B3), folate, vitamin C, and vegetable protein. They are higher in calcium than most vegetables and also contain good levels of magnesium, iron, zinc, and potassium.

- Very high in fiber and soluble fiber to help lower "bad" blood cholesterol.
- Quercetin, magnesium, and vitamin C content protect the heart.
- Very good source of a range of important minerals.
- May help liver and gall bladder function.

Practical tips:
Fresh pods should be bright green and firm. Limp pods or those with brown patches are past their best. The beans should be harvested when they are small so that you can eat the fiber-rich outer skin of each bean. Very young beans can be eaten raw. Older beans are best with this skin removed and cooked by steaming to retain most of the vitamin C and niacin content.

DID YOU KNOW?

Fava beans contain L-dopa, a chemical that helps produce dopamine in the body, which is the neurotransmitter associated with the "feel good" factor in the brain.

MAJOR NUTRIENTS PER 3½ oz/100 G SHELLED FAVA BEANS

Kcalories	81
Total fat	0.6 g
Protein	8 g
Carbohydrate	11.7 g
Fiber	6.5 g
Vitamin C	8 mg
Folate	32 mcg
Niacin	3.0 mg
Beta-carotene	225 mcg
Magnesium	36 mg
Potassium	280 mg
Iron	1.6 mg
Calcium	56 mg
Zinc	1.0 mg

Fava bean salad

SERVES 4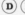

*5 lb 8 oz/2.5 kg fresh fava beans in
the pod, shelled or 15 oz/425 g
frozen fava beans*

*2 tomatoes, peeled, seeded,
and diced*

3 tbsp shredded fresh basil

*4 level tbsp fresh Parmesan cheese
shavings*

Dressing

1 tsp white wine vinegar

1 small garlic clove, crushed

4 tbsp extra virgin olive oil

salt and pepper

Method

1 Cook the fava beans in a large
saucepan of boiling water for
3 minutes, or until just tender.
Drain and tip into a large
serving dish or arrange on
4 serving plates.

2 Whisk the dressing ingredients
together in a bowl or pitcher
and spoon over the beans
while they are still warm.

3 Scatter over the diced tomato,
basil, and Parmesan shavings.
Serve at room temperature.

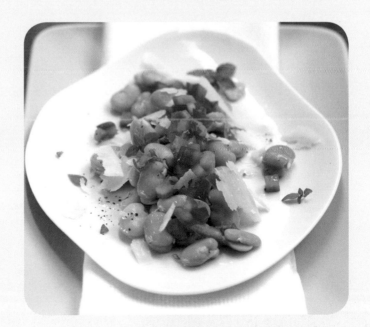

26 TOMATOES

The tomato is one of the healthiest salad foods because it contains lycopene, which offers protection from prostate cancer, and compounds to help prevent blood clots.

Tomatoes are our major source of dietary lycopene, a carotene antioxidant that fights heart disease and may help to prevent prostate cancer. Tomatoes also have an anticoagulant effect because of the salicylates contained in them, and they contain several other antioxidants including vitamin C, quercetin, and lutein. Tomatoes are low in calories but high in potassium, and contain useful amounts of fiber.

- Excellent source of lycopene, which helps prevent prostate cancer.
- One medium tomato contains nearly a quarter of the day's recommended intake of vitamin C for an adult.
- Rich in potassium to help regulate body fluids.
- Quercetin and lutein content helps to prevent cataracts and keep heart and eyes healthy.
- Contain salicylates, which have an anticoagulant effect.

Practical tips:
The more red and ripe the tomato is, the higher its content of lycopene. Vine-ripened tomatoes also contain more lycopene than those ripened after picking. The tomato peel is richer in nutrients than the flesh and the central seed part is high in salicylates, so avoid peeling and don't seed unless necessary. The lycopene in raw or cooked tomatoes is better absorbed in your body if it is eaten with some oil, such as a salad dressing.

DID YOU KNOW?

Lycopene is actually more active in processed tomato products such as ketchup, tomato paste, and tomato juice than it is in the raw tomato.

MAJOR NUTRIENTS PER 3½ oz/100 g TOMATO

Kcalories	18
Total fat	0.2 g
Protein	0.9 g
Carbohydrate	3.9 g
Fiber	1.2 g
Vitamin C	12.7 mg
Potassium	237 mg
Lycopene	2573 mcg
Lutein/Zeaxanthin	123 mcg

Tomato sauce

MAKES ABOUT 2½ CUPS (V) (D) (P) (C)

1 tbsp olive oil

1 small onion, chopped

2–3 garlic cloves, crushed
  (optional)

1 small celery stalk, finely chopped

1 bay leaf

1 lb/450 g ripe tomatoes, peeled
  and chopped

1 tbsp tomato paste, blended with
  ⅔ cup water

few fresh oregano sprigs

pepper

Method

1 Heat the oil in a heavy-bottom saucepan. Add the onion, garlic, if using, celery, and bay leaf, and gently sauté, stirring frequently, for 5 minutes.

2 Stir in the tomatoes with the blended tomato paste. Season with pepper to taste and add the oregano. Bring to a boil, then reduce the heat, cover, and simmer, stirring occasionally, for 20–25 minutes, until the tomatoes have completely collapsed. If liked, simmer for an additional 20 minutes to give a thicker sauce.

3 Discard the bay leaf and the oregano. Transfer to a food processor and process until a chunky puree forms. If a smooth sauce is preferred, pass through a fine nonmetallic strainer. Taste and adjust the seasoning, if necessary. Reheat and use as required.

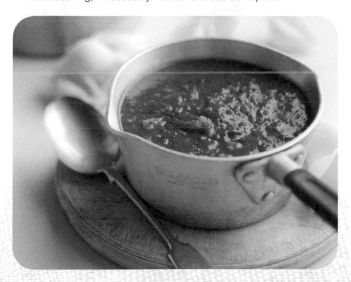

27 SPINACH

Contrary to popular belief, spinach doesn't contain as much iron as originally thought but, nevertheless, it has many excellent health benefits.

Researchers have found many flavonoid compounds in spinach act as antioxidants and fight against stomach, skin, breast, prostate, and other cancers. Spinach is also extremely high in carotenes, which protect eyesight. It is also particularly rich in vitamin K, which helps to boost bone strength and may help prevent osteoporosis. In addition, spinach also contains peptides, which are aspects of protein that have been shown to lower blood pressure, and its relatively high vitamin E content may help protect the brain from cognitive decline as we age.

- Flavonoid and carotene content protects against many cancers.
- Vitamin C, folate, and carotene content helps maintain artery health and prevent atherosclerosis.
- Helps keep eyes healthy.
- Vitamin K content boosts bone density.

Practical tips:
Avoid buying spinach with any yellowing leaves. The carotenes in spinach are better absorbed when the leaves are cooked rather than eaten raw, and also if eaten with a little oil. Steaming or stir-frying retains the most antioxidants. To cook, simply wash the leaves and cook in only the water still clinging to the leaves, stirring if necessary.

DID YOU KNOW?

Researchers found that feeding aging laboratory animals spinach-rich diets significantly improved both their learning capacity and motor skills.

MAJOR NUTRIENTS PER 3½ oz/100 G SPINACH

Kcalories	23
Total fat	0.4 g
Protein	2.9 g
Carbohydrate	3.6 g
Fiber	2.2 g
Vitamin C	28 mg
Folate	194 mcg
Vitamin E	2 mg
Vitamin K	482 mcg
Potassium	558 mg
Magnesium	79 mg
Calcium	99 mg
Iron	2.7 mg
Beta-carotene	5,626 mcg
Lutein/Zeaxanthin	12,198 mcg

Red curry with mixed leaves

SERVES 4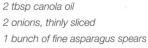

2 tbsp canola oil

2 onions, thinly sliced

1 bunch of fine asparagus spears

1¾ cups low-fat coconut milk

2 tbsp red curry paste

3 fresh kaffir lime leaves

8 oz/225 g baby spinach leaves

2 heads bok choy, chopped

1 small head Chinese cabbage,
    shredded

handful of fresh cilantro, chopped

cooked rice, to serve

Method

1 Heat a large wok over medium–high heat for 30 seconds. Add the oil, swirl it around to coat the bottom, and heat for 30 seconds. Add the onions and asparagus and stir-fry for 1–2 minutes.

2 Add the coconut milk, curry paste, and lime leaves and bring gently to a boil. Add the spinach, bok choy, and cabbage and cook for 2–3 minutes, until wilted. Stir in the cilantro and serve with rice.

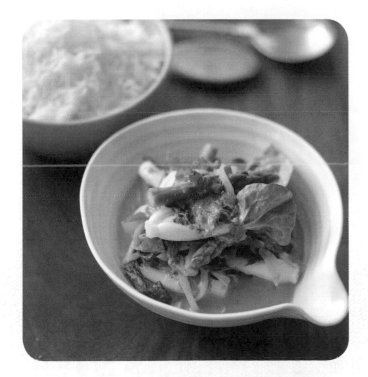

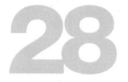

GARLIC

Valued as a health-protector for thousands of years, garlic bulbs are a useful antibiotic, and can also reduce the risk of both heart disease and cancer.

Although often used only in small quantities, garlic can still make an impact on health. It is rich in powerful sulfur compounds that cause garlic's strong odor but are the main source of its health benefits. Research has found that garlic can help minimize the risk of both heart disease and many types of cancer. It is also a powerful antibiotic and inhibits fungal infections such as athlete's foot. It also appears to minimize stomach ulcers. Eaten in reasonable quantity, it is also a good source of vitamin C, selenium, potassium, and calcium. Garlic should be crushed or chopped and allowed to stand for a few minutes before cooking.

- May prevent formation of blood clots and arterial plaque and help prevent heart disease.
- Regular garlic consumption may significantly reduce the risk of colon, stomach, and prostate cancer.
- Natural antibiotic, antiviral, and antifungal.
- Can help prevent stomach ulcers.

Practical tips:
Choose large, firm, undamaged bulbs and store in a container with air holes, in a dark, cool, dry, place. Skin the garlic by lightly crushing the clove with the flat side of a cleaver or knife and only lightly cook—long cooking destroys its beneficial compounds. Parsley eaten after a garlic meal may reduce any mouth odor.

DID YOU KNOW?

Meat cooked at high temperatures, such as broiling or barbecuing, can have a carcinogenic effect, but when garlic is used with the meat it reduces the production of the cancer-promoting chemicals.

MAJOR NUTRIENTS PER 2 GARLIC CLOVES

Kcalories	9
Total fat	Trace
Protein	0.4 g
Carbohydrate	2 g
Fiber	Trace
Vitamin C	2 mg
Potassium	24 mg
Calcium	11 mg
Selenium	1 mcg

Mushrooms with roasted garlic and scallions

SERVES 4

2 garlic bulbs

2 tbsp olive oil

*12 oz/350 g assorted mushrooms,
such as cremini, open-cap, and
chanterelles, halved if large*

1 tbsp chopped fresh parsley

*8 scallions, cut into
1-inch/2.5-cm lengths*

salt and pepper

Method

1 Preheat the oven to
350°F/180°C. Slice off the
tops of the garlic bulbs and
press down to loosen the
cloves. Place them in an
ovenproof dish and season
with salt and pepper to taste.
Drizzle 2 teaspoons of the oil
over the bulbs and roast
for 30 minutes. Remove the
garlic from the oven and
drizzle with 1 teaspoon of the
remaining oil. Return to the
oven and roast for an
additional 45 minutes. Remove
the garlic from the oven and
leave until cool enough to
handle, then peel the cloves.

2 Tip the oil from the dish into a
heavy-bottom skillet. Add the
remaining oil and heat. Add
the mushrooms and cook over
medium heat, stirring
frequently, for 4 minutes.

3 Add the garlic cloves, parsley,
and scallions and cook, stirring
frequently, for 5 minutes.
Season with salt and pepper
to taste and serve immediately.

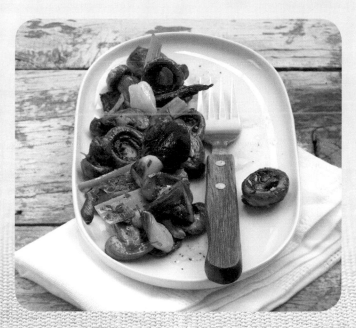

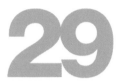

ARTICHOKES

Globe artichokes are low in calories and ideal for dieters, and their cynarin content helps maintain liver health.

A delicious delicacy, globe artichokes are the unopened flowers of a large perennial plant. The whole vegetable can be served as an appetizer, but only the tender leaf bases and more nutritious central heart are edible. Artichokes are one of the richest vegetable sources of a range of minerals, including calcium, iron, magnesium, and potassium. They are also very high in fiber, and contain a compound called cynarin that is said to boost liver function.

- Very rich source of minerals including calcium, iron, and the antioxidant mineral magnesium for bone and heart health.
- Very high in fiber with a high proportion of soluble fiber for healthy blood cholesterol.
- Good source of vitamin C and folate.
- Low in calories and low on the glycemic index.

Practical tips:
Very small baby artichokes can be eaten whole but, for larger ones, snap off the stem, cut off the top third of the artichoke, and remove the tough outer leaves individually by hand. Simmer in boiling water containing a little lemon juice for 20 minutes, or until the leaves are easy to remove. Eat only the creamy bases of each leaf. Once the leaves are removed, the bristly choke should be pulled out to reveal the tender heart, which is delicious served hot with a dressing, cold in a salad, or with pasta.

DID YOU KNOW?

Iron, copper, and aluminum cookware will cause artichokes to oxidize and discolor, so use stainless steel, glass, or enamel.

MAJOR NUTRIENTS PER AVERAGE-SIZED ARTICHOKE

Kcalories	60
Total fat	trace
Protein	4.2 g
Carbohydrate	13.4 g
Fiber	6.5 g
Vitamin C	12 mg
Folate	65 mcg
Potassium	425 mg
Magnesium	72 mg
Calcium	54 mg
Iron	1.5 mg
Lutein/Zeaxanthin	557 mcg

Artichoke hearts and asparagus

SERVES 4–6

1 lb/450 g asparagus spears
14 oz/400 g canned artichoke
  hearts, drained and rinsed
salad greens, to serve

Dressing

2 tbsp freshly squeezed
  orange juice
½ tsp finely grated orange rind
2 tbsp walnut oil
1 tsp Dijon mustard
salt and pepper

Method

1 Trim and discard the coarse, woody ends of the asparagus spears. Make sure all the stems are the same length, then tie them together loosely with clean kitchen string. If you have an asparagus steamer, you don't need to tie the stems together—just place them in the basket.

2 Cook the asparagus in a tall saucepan of lightly salted, boiling water over medium heat for 5 minutes, or until tender. Make sure that the tips protrude above the water. Drain, then refresh under cold running water and drain again.

3 Cut the asparagus spears into 1-inch/2.5-cm pieces, keeping the tips intact. Cut the artichoke hearts into small wedges and combine with the asparagus in a bowl.

4 Whisk the orange juice, orange rind, walnut oil, and mustard together in a bowl and season with salt and pepper to taste. If serving immediately, pour the dressing over the artichoke hearts and asparagus and toss lightly.

5 To serve, arrange the salad greens in individual serving dishes and top with the artichoke and asparagus mixture.

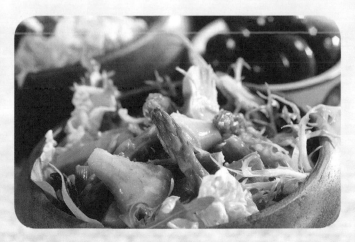

30

FENNEL

Bulbs of fennel are rich in a variety of antioxidants, which can reduce inflammation and help to prevent cancer.

Fennel is grown for its thick, crunchy bulbous base. It is refreshing, slightly sweet, and contains a strong anise flavor. Fennel contains a potent combination of plant chemicals, which give it strong antioxidant activity. One of the most interesting compounds in fennel is anethole. In animal studies, the anethole in fennel has been shown to reduce inflammation and to help prevent the occurrence of cancer. It is also a very good source of fiber, folate, and potassium, and contains a wide range of other nutrients including vitamin C, selenium, niacin (vitamin B3), and iron. The very high potassium content means that fennel is a diuretic, helping to eliminate surplus fluid from the body.

• Diuretic, digestive aid, and antiflatulent.
• Very low in calories, making it an ideal food for dieters.
• Anti-inflammatory.
• Rich in antioxidant compounds for disease prevention.

Practical tips:
Choose bulbs that are firm and solid with a slight gloss and healthy looking leaf tops. Store in the refrigerator—fennel bulbs lose their flavor after a few days. Fennel is delicious thinly sliced raw in salads and goes particularly well with fish. Try baking small whole fish in aluminum foil, on a bed of thinly sliced fennel. Fennel can also be quartered, browned in oil then braised with a little vegetable stock.

DID YOU KNOW?

Fennel is closely related to the fennel herb and the leafy tops of the bulb can be chopped and used in a similar way to the herb.

MAJOR NUTRIENTS PER HALF FENNEL BULB

Kcalories	12
Total fat	Trace
Protein	0.9 g
Carbohydrate	1.8 g
Fiber	2.4 g
Vitamin C	5 mg
Folate	42 mcg
Beta-carotene	140 mg
Calcium	24 mg
Potassium	440 mg
Selenium	0.7 mcg

Fennel and orange salad

SERVES 4

2 oranges, peeled and sliced
1 bulb Florence fennel,
    thinly sliced, plus fennel fronds,
    to garnish
1 red onion, sliced into thin rings
pepper

Dressing

juice of 1 orange
2 tbsp balsamic vinegar

Method

1 Arrange the orange slices in the bottom of a shallow dish. Place a layer of fennel on top and then add a layer of onion.
2 Mix the orange juice and vinegar together and drizzle over the salad. Season with pepper, garnish with fennel fronds, and serve.

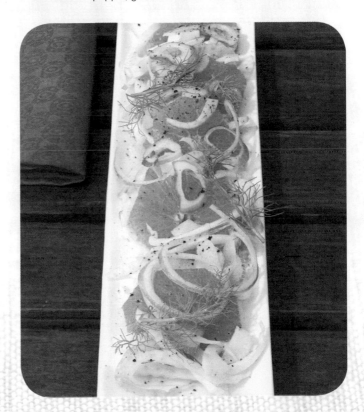

31 KALE

Deep green kale contains the highest levels of antioxidants of all vegetables and is a very good source of vitamin C.

Kale is one of the most nutritious members of the brassica family. It rates as the vegetable highest in antioxidant capacity on the ORAC scale, and contains more calcium and iron than any other vegetable. A single portion contains twice the recommended daily amount of vitamin C, which helps the vegetable's high iron content to be absorbed in our bodies. One portion also gives about a fifth of the daily calcium requirement for an adult. Kale is rich in selenium, which helps fight cancer, and it contains magnesium and vitamin E for a healthy heart. The range of nutrients kale provides will keep skin young looking and healthy.

- Rich in flavonoids and antioxidants to fight cancers.
- Contains indoles, which can help lower "bad" cholesterol and prevent cancer.
- Calcium rich for healthy bones.
- Extremely rich in carotenes to protect eyes.

Practical tips:
Wash kale before use as the curly leaves may contain sand or soil. Don't discard the outer, deep green leaves—these contain rich amounts of carotenes and indoles. Kale is good steamed or stir-fried and its strong taste goes well with bacon, eggs, and cheese. Kale, like spinach, shrinks a lot during cooking, so make sure you add plenty to the pan.

DID YOU KNOW?

Kale contains naturally occurring substances that can interfere with the functioning of the thyroid gland—those with thyroid problems may not want to eat kale.

MAJOR NUTRIENTS PER 3½ oz/100 g KALE

Kcalories	50
Total fat	0.7 g
Protein	3.3 g
Carbohydrate	10 g
Fiber	2 g
Vitamin C	120 mg
Folate	29 mcg
Vitamin E	1.7 mg
Potassium	447 mg
Magnesium	34 mg
Calcium	135 mg
Iron	1.7 mg
Selenium	0.9 mcg
Beta-carotene	9226 mcg
Lutein/Zeaxanthin	39550 mcg

Kale stir-fry

SERVES 4

1 lb 10 oz/750 g fresh kale
2 tbsp canola oil
1 onion, chopped
4 large garlic cloves, finely chopped
2 red bell peppers, thinly sliced
1 carrot, peeled and grated
3½ oz/100 g tiny broccoli florets
pinch of dried chili flakes (optional)
½ cup vegetable stock
4 oz/115 g fresh bean sprouts
salt and pepper
*handful of chopped toasted
    cashews, to garnish*
*cooked rice and lemon wedges,
    to serve*

Method

1 Using a sharp knife, remove any thick central cores from the kale. Stack several leaves on top of each other, then cut across them into fine shreds; repeat until all the kale is shredded. Set aside.

2 Heat a large wok or saucepan with a lid over high heat for 30 seconds. Add the oil, swirl it around to coat the bottom, and heat for 30 seconds. Add the onion and stir-fry for about 3 minutes, then add the garlic, bell peppers, and carrot and continue stir-frying until the onion is tender and the bell peppers are starting to soften. Add the broccoli and chili flakes, if using, and stir.

3 Add the kale to the wok and stir, then add the stock and salt and pepper to taste. Reduce the heat to medium, cover, and simmer for about 5 minutes, until the kale is tender.

4 Remove the lid and allow any excess liquid to evaporate. Use 2 forks to mix the bean sprouts through the other ingredients, then adjust the seasoning, if necessary. Serve the vegetables on a bed of rice, with cashews sprinkled over, and lemon wedges on the side for squeezing over.

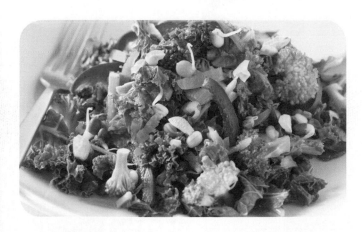

32 CELERY

High in potassium and calcium, celery helps to reduce fluid retention and prevent high blood pressure.

Celery has long been regarded as an ideal food for dieters because of its high water content and therefore its low calorie content. In fact, celery is a useful and healthy vegetable for many other reasons. It is a good source of potassium and is also surprisingly high in calcium, vital for healthy bones, healthy blood pressure levels, and nerve function. The darker green stalks and the leaves of celery contain carotenes and more of the minerals and vitamin C than the paler leaves, so don't discard them. Celery also contains the compounds polyacetalines and phthalides, which may protect us from inflammation and high blood pressure.

- Low in calories and fat and high in fiber.
- Good source of potassium.
- Calcium content protects bones and may help regulate blood pressure.
- May offer protection from inflammation.

Practical tips:
Choose celery heads with leaves that look bright green and fresh. Store in a plastic bag or in plastic wrap to prevent the stalks going limp. Celery is ideal for adding flavor and bulk to soups and stews and quartered heads can be braised in vegetable stock for an excellent accompaniment to fish, poultry, or game. The leaves can be added to salads and stir-fries or used as a garnish.

DID YOU KNOW?

Celery can contain high levels of nitrates, which have been linked with an increased risk of cancer. However, research has found that vegetables high in nitrates also usually contain high levels of nitrate-neutralizing chemicals.

MAJOR NUTRIENTS PER 3½ oz/100 G CELERY STALK

Kcalories	14
Total fat	Trace
Protein	0.7 g
Carbohydrate	3 g
Fiber	1.6 g
Vitamin C	3 mg
Folate	36 mcg
Vitamin K	35 mcg
Potassium	260 mg
Calcium	40 mg
Magnesium	11 mg

Celery and apple revitalizer

SERVES 2

4 oz/115 g celery, chopped
1 apple, peeled, cored,
    and diced
2½ cups milk
pinch of sugar (optional)
salt (optional)
strips of celery, for decorating

Method

1 Place the celery, apple, and milk in a blender and process until thoroughly combined.

2 Stir in the sugar and some salt, if using. Pour into chilled glasses, decorate with strips of celery, and serve.

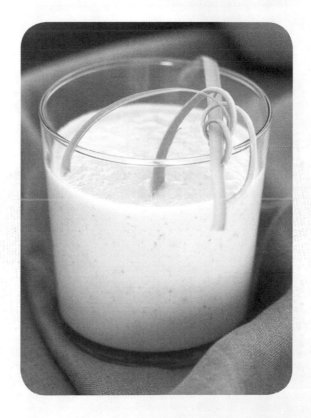

33 ASPARAGUS

The distinctive asparagus is an anti-inflammatory and contains a type of fiber that keeps the digestive system healthy.

The plant chemical glutathione contained in asparagus has been found to be anti-inflammatory and may help rheumatoid arthritis symptoms. The vegetable is also rich in the soluble fiber oligosaccharide, which acts as a prebiotic in the gut by stimulating the growth of "friendly" bacteria. It is also a valuable source of vitamin C, folate, magnesium, potassium, and iron. Unusually for a vegetable, it is a good source of vitamin E, an antioxidant that helps keep the heart and immune system healthy.

- Glutathione content is anti-inflammatory.
- Fiber content acts as a prebiotic for gut health.
- Good source of a wide range of important vitamins, including vitamin E.
- Rich in iron, promotes energy and healing, and helps fights infection.

DID YOU KNOW?
Asparagus contains purines, compounds that encourage the production of uric acid in the body, which can trigger an attack of gout. Gout sufferers should avoid asparagus, or only consume it in moderation.

MAJOR NUTRIENTS PER 10 ASPARAGUS SPEARS

Kcalories	24
Total fat	Trace
Protein	2.6 g
Carbohydrate	4.7 g
Fiber	2.5 g
Vitamin C	6.7 mg
Vitamin E	1.36 mg
Folate	62 mcg
Potassium	242 mg
Calcium	29 mg
Magnesium	17 mg
Iron	2.6 mg

Practical tips:
Asparagus doesn't store well and should be eaten as soon as possible after picking. If necessary, store in a plastic bag in the refrigerator for one to two days. If possible, cook the spears upright in a pan so that the delicate tips don't overcook before the stalks are tender. Large spears can also be brushed with oil and broiled for 2–3 minutes a side, until tender. Small, thin asparagus spears can be used in quiches, soups, and risottos.

Asparagus with sweet tomato dressing

SERVES 4

5 tbsp extra virgin olive oil, plus
   extra for brushing
½ cup pine nuts
1 lb 2 oz/500 g young asparagus
   spears, trimmed
1 oz/25 g Parmesan cheese,
   thinly shaved

Dressing

12 oz/350 g tomatoes, peeled,
   seeded, and chopped
2 tbsp balsamic vinegar
salt and pepper

Method

1 Brush the broiler rack with oil and preheat the broiler to high. Heat
  a nonstick skillet over medium heat. Add the pine nuts and lightly
  toast until just browned. Tip into a bowl and set aside.

2 Next, make the dressing by mixing the tomatoes, vinegar, and
  olive oil together in a bowl and season with salt and pepper to taste.
  Set aside.

3 Arrange the asparagus spears on the broiler rack and cook under
  the preheated broiler for 3–4 minutes until tender. Carefully transfer
  to a serving dish. Spoon over the dressing, sprinkle with the pine
  nuts and Parmesan cheese shavings, and serve immediately.

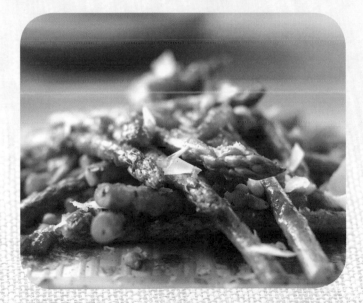

34 PEAS

Either freshly picked or bought frozen, peas are a rich source of vitamin C, fiber, protein, and lutein for eye health.

Peas are rich in a wide range of useful vitamins and minerals. They are particularly high in antioxidant vitamin C, folate, and vitamin B3, and their very high lutein and zeaxanthin content means that they help protect the eyes from macular degeneration. The B vitamins they contain may also help protect the bones from osteoporosis, and help to decrease the risk of strokes by keeping levels of the amino acid homocysteine low in the blood. Peas, high in protein, are very useful for vegetarians. In addition, their high fiber content partly comprises pectin, a jellylike substance that helps to lower "bad" blood cholesterol and may also help prevent heart and arterial disease.

- Contain several heart-friendly nutrients and chemicals.
- Rich in carotenes to protect eyes and reduce risk of cancers.
- Very high in total and soluble fiber to lower cholesterol.
- Very rich in vitamin C.

Practical tips:
When buying peas in the pod choose those that aren't packed in too tightly. Older peas become almost square, lose their flavor, and become mealy because the sugars have been converted to starches. Young pods can be eaten with the peas inside and young peas can be eaten raw. To cook, steam lightly or boil in minimal water, as the vitamin C content leaches into the water.

DID YOU KNOW?

Frozen peas—usually frozen within hours of harvesting—can often contain more vitamin C and other nutrients than fresh peas in their pods, which may be several days old.

MAJOR NUTRIENTS PER 3½ oz/100 g SHELLED PEAS

Kcalories	81
Total fat	0.4 g
Protein	5.4 g
Carbohydrate	14.5 g
Fiber	5.1 g
Vitamin C	40 mg
Folate	65 mcg
Niacin	2.1 mg
Magnesium	33 mg
Potassium	244 mg
Iron	1.5 mg
Calcium	56 mg
Zinc	1.2 mg
Lutein/Zeaxanthin	2477 mcg

Chilled pea soup

SERVES 3–4

generous 1¾ cups vegetable stock
  or water
4½ cups frozen peas
2 oz/55 g scallions, coarsely
  chopped
1¼ cups plain yogurt
salt and pepper

To garnish
2 tbsp chopped fresh mint
2 tbsp chopped scallions or chives
grated lemon rind
olive oil

Method

1 Bring the stock to a boil in a large saucepan over medium heat. Reduce the heat, add the peas and scallions, and simmer for 5 minutes.

2 Let cool slightly, then strain twice, making sure that you remove any bits of skin. Pour into a large bowl, season with salt and pepper to taste, and stir in the yogurt. Cover the bowl with plastic wrap and chill in the refrigerator for several hours, or until well chilled.

3 To serve, remove from the refrigerator, mix well, and ladle into soup bowls. Garnish with the chopped mint, scallions, grated lemon rind, and olive oil.

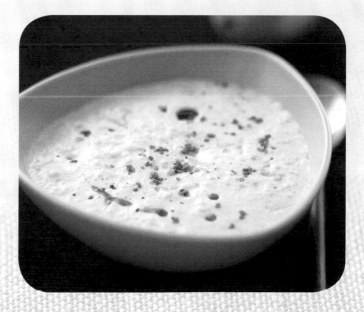

35 BEETS

This colorful, sweet root may not be the richest vegetable in nutrients but it certainly should not be overlooked and is invaluable during the winter season.

Beet comes in white and gold varieties as well as the classic purple-red, which is the best source of nutrients. Betaine, which gives it its deep color, is even more potent an antioxidant than polyphenols in its effect on lowering blood pressure. A scientific study also found that the high levels of nitrates in beet juice work like aspirin to prevent blood clots, and help to protect the lining of the blood vessels. Red beet is also rich in anthocyanins, which may help to prevent colon and other cancers.

- Contain betaine to lower blood pressure and may be anti-inflammatory.
- Contain nitrates to help prevent blood clots.
- Anthocyanins can help prevent cancers.
- A good source of iron, magnesium, and folate.

DID YOU KNOW?

Beets were originally cultivated for their nutritious leaves, which can still be eaten when small, in the same way as spinach.

MAJOR NUTRIENTS PER 3½ oz/100 G BEETS

Kcalories	36
Total fat	Trace
Protein	1.7 g
Carbohydrate	7.6 g
Fiber	1.9 g
Vitamin C	5 mg
Folate	150 mcg
Potassium	380 mg
Calcium	20 mg
Iron	1.0 mg
Magnesium	23 mg

Practical tips:

Cooked beets will keep in an airtight container for a few days in the refrigerator or you can puree cooked beets and freeze. To cook, cut off the leaves but leave about 2 inches/5 cm of stalk and the root still on. This will avoid the beet "bleeding" as it cooks. Beets can be boiled whole for about 50 minutes or brushed with a little oil and baked in aluminum foil at 400°F/200°C for 1 hour. The skins can then be easily rubbed off. Beet can also be used raw, peeled, and finely grated into salads or salsa, or juiced.

Beet and spinach salad

SERVES 4

1 lb 7 oz/650 g cooked beets
3 tbsp extra virgin olive oil
juice of 1 orange
1 tsp superfine sugar
1 tsp fennel seeds
4 oz/115 g fresh baby spinach
   leaves
salt and pepper

Method

1 Using a sharp knife, dice the cooked beets and set aside until required. Heat the olive oil in a small, heavy-bottom saucepan. Add the orange juice, sugar, and fennel seeds and season with salt and pepper to taste. Stir continuously until the sugar has dissolved.

2 Add the beets to the saucepan and stir gently to coat. Remove from the heat.

3 Arrange the baby spinach leaves in a large salad bowl. Spoon the warmed beets on top and serve immediately.

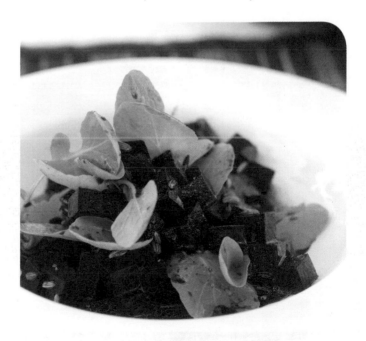

36 RED CABBAGE

This vegetable is rich in compounds that protect us from cancers and the signs of aging.

A member of the brassica family, purple-red cabbage is high in nutrients and contains protective plant compounds. These include: indoles, which have been linked with protection against hormone-based cancers such as breast, uterus, and ovarian; sulphorophane, which can help block cancer-causing chemicals; and monoterpenes, which protect body cells from damage by free radicals. Red cabbage is much higher in immunity boosting carotenes than other cabbages—lycopene is linked with protection from prostate cancer, and anthocyanins may protect against Alzheimer's disease. The red cabbage is also higher in vitamin C than pale varieties and is a good source of minerals, including calcium and selenium.

- Contains a variety of cancer-fighting compounds.
- Low in calories, with a low glycemic index—ideal for dieters.
- Rich in the antioxidant vitamin C.
- Anthocyanin content may protect against Alzheimer's disease.

Practical tips:
Thinly sliced red cabbage can be used raw in coleslaw instead of white cabbage. Sprinkle with lemon juice or salad dressing to prevent it from turning gray. Once cut, red cabbage should be used within one to two days. When cooking, steaming preserves the maximum nutrients, so try not to overcook.

DID YOU KNOW?

Cabbage leaves have natural antiseptic properties and can be applied directly to wounds and bruises to help relieve pain and healing.

MAJOR NUTRIENTS PER 3½ oz/100 G RED CABBAGE

Kcalories	31
Total fat	trace
Protein	1.4 g
Carbohydrate	7.4 g
Fiber	2.1 g
Vitamin C	57 mg
Folate	18 mcg
Niacin	0.4 mg
Potassium	243 mg
Iron	0.8 mg
Calcium	45 mg
Selenium	0.6 mcg
Beta-carotene	670 mg
Lutein/Zeaxanthin	329 mcg

Cabbage and walnut stir-fry

SERVES 4

12 oz/350 g white cabbage
12 oz/350 g red cabbage
4 tbsp peanut oil
1 tbsp walnut oil
2 garlic cloves, crushed
8 scallions, trimmed
8 oz/225 g firm tofu, cubed
2 tbsp lemon juice
1 cup walnut halves
2 tsp Dijon mustard
salt and pepper
2 tsp poppy seeds, to garnish

Method

1 Using a sharp knife, thinly shred the white and red cabbages and set aside until needed.
2 Heat a wok over high heat for 30 seconds. Add the oils, swirl them around to coat the bottom, and heat for an additional 30 seconds. Add the garlic, cabbage, scallions, and tofu and stir-fry for 5 minutes.
3 Add the lemon juice, walnuts, and mustard to the wok and stir to combine thoroughly. Season with salt and pepper to taste and cook for an additional 5 minutes, or until the cabbage is tender.
4 Transfer the stir-fry to a warmed serving bowl, sprinkle with poppy seeds, and serve immediately.

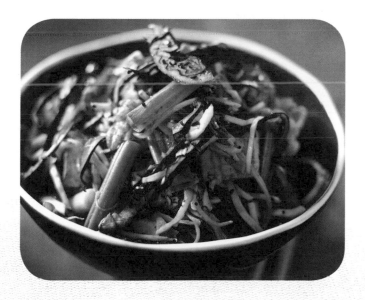

37

SEAWEED

Rich in iodine for healthy thyroid action, zinc for fertility, and calcium for healthy bones, seaweed is highly nutritious.

While there are thousands of different varieties of seaweed, only a few are widely available or commonly used as a vegetable. Often found dried, the most well known are flat, dark green kelp (also known as kombu), dark red dulse, green or purple nori, and dark green or brown wakame. The nutritional value of the types varies but they are mostly rich in iron, calcium, zinc, magnesium, and iodine, a mineral that can help to boost the action of the thyroid gland, regulate the body's metabolism, and help hearing. Seaweed is also rich in folate and low in calories.

- Rich in easily absorbed minerals and ideal for vegetarians.
- Good food for dieters as seaweed is low in calories and contains a gel-like substance called agar, which helps you to feel full for longer.
- May be antiviral and anticancer.
- Excellent source of iodine to help the body's metabolism.

Practical tips:
Fresh seaweed for consumption should be sourced from unpolluted waters. It can be chopped and used in soups or stir-fried as a garnish. Laver, a type of seaweed, is used in parts of the UK to make a flat bread that is shallow fried. Dried seaweed can be reconstituted according to the package directions and used in a similar way. Large sheets of nori are used to wrap sushi.

DID YOU KNOW?

Most types of seaweed are high in sodium (because the sea is very salty) and therefore not suitable for anyone on a low-sodium diet.

MAJOR NUTRIENTS PER 1¾ oz/50 G KELP

Kcalories	22
Total fat	0.3 g
Protein	0.8 g
Carbohydrate	4.8 g
Fiber	0.7 g
Calcium	84 mg
Iron	1.4 mg
Magnesium	61 mg
Potassium	45 mg
Zinc	.06 mg
Iodine	1037 mcg
Folate	90 mcg

Mixed sushi

SERVES 4 (D)(C)

scant 1¼ cups sushi rice
2 tbsp rice vinegar
1 tsp superfine sugar
½ tsp salt
4 sheets nori (seaweed), for rolling
1¾ oz/50 g smoked salmon
1½-inch/4-cm piece cucumber,
  peeled, seeded, and cut into
  matchsticks
1½ oz/40 g cooked peeled shrimp
1 small avocado, pitted, peeled,
  thinly sliced, and tossed in
  lemon juice

To serve
wasabi
tamari
pink pickled ginger

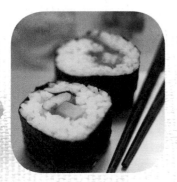

Method

1 Place the rice in a saucepan and cover with cold water. Bring to a boil, then reduce the heat, cover, and simmer for 15–20 minutes, or until the rice is tender and the water has been absorbed. Drain if necessary and transfer to a bowl. Mix the vinegar, sugar, and salt together, then, using a spatula, stir well into the rice. Cover with a damp cloth and let cool.

2 To make the rolls, lay a clean bamboo mat over a cutting board. Lay a sheet of nori, shiny side-down, on the mat. Spread a quarter of the rice mixture over the nori, using wet fingers to press it down evenly, leaving a ½-inch/1-cm margin at the top and bottom.

3 For smoked salmon and cucumber rolls, lay the salmon over the rice and arrange the cucumber in a line across the center. For the shrimp rolls, lay the shrimp and avocado in a line across the center.

4 Carefully hold the nearest edge of the mat, then, using the mat as a guide, roll up the nori tightly to make a neat tube of rice enclosing the filling. Seal the uncovered edge with a little water, then roll the sushi off the mat. Repeat to make 3 more rolls —you need 2 salmon and cucumber and 2 shrimp and avocado in total.

5 Using a wet knife, cut each roll into 8 pieces and stand upright on a platter. Wipe and rinse the knife between cuts to prevent the rice from sticking. Serve the rolls with wasabi, tamari, and pickled ginger.

38 MUSHROOMS

The compounds in mushrooms, which boost the immune system, help to prevent cancers, infections, and auto-immune diseases such as arthritis and lupus.

Most of the mushrooms that we buy are the young, white-skinned button mushrooms and the older, darker gilled flat mushrooms, but there are several others, such as Chinese shiitake mushrooms, Italian porcini, and wild mushrooms. While the amount of beneficial compounds varies according to their variety and age, (older, darker ones have more benefits), most mushrooms are rich in plant chemicals, which help boost the immune system. An active component of mushrooms that may be beneficial is glutamic acid, a naturally occurring form of monosodium glutamate. Mushrooms are also a useful source of protein.

- Contain compounds that can help prevent cancers and auto-immune diseases.
- Ideal source of healthy protein for vegetarians and dieters.
- Rich in the anticancer antioxidant mineral selenium.
- Good source of B vitamins, including folate and niacin, which has cholesterol-lowering properties.

Practical tips:
Store mushrooms in the refrigerator in a paper bag rather than a plastic bag, to help them breathe. Most mushrooms shouldn't need washing but if any compost clings to them, gently wipe with paper towels. Don't peel or remove the stalks—these contain much of their goodness.

DID YOU KNOW?

You should not pick mushrooms from the wild unless you get them checked for safety by a fungi expert. Several varieties look harmless but are poisonous.

MAJOR NUTRIENTS PER 3 oz/85 G MUSHROOMS

Kcalories	22
Total fat	Trace
Protein	2.1 g
Carbohydrate	4.2 g
Fiber	1.3 g
Niacin (Vitamin B3)	3.8 mg
Folate	18 mcg
Calcium	7 mg
Iron	0.5 mg
Potassium	407 mg
Selenium	9.2 mcg
Zinc	0.5 mg

Mixed mushroom salad

SERVES 4

3 tbsp pine nuts
2 red onions, chopped
4 tbsp olive oil
2 garlic cloves, crushed
3 slices whole wheat bread, cubed
7 oz/200 g mixed salad greens
9 oz/250 g cremini mushrooms,
    sliced
5½ oz/150 g shiitake mushrooms,
    sliced
5½ oz/150 g oyster mushrooms,
    torn

Dressing

1 garlic clove, crushed
2 tbsp red wine vinegar
4 tbsp walnut oil
1 tbsp finely chopped fresh
    parsley
pepper

Method

1 Preheat the oven to 350°F/180°C. Heat a nonstick skillet over medium heat. Add the pine nuts and lightly toast until just browned. Tip into a bowl and set aside.

2 Place the onions and 1 tablespoon of the oil in a roasting pan and toss to coat. Roast in the preheated oven for 30 minutes.

3 Meanwhile, heat 1 tablespoon of the remaining oil with the garlic in the skillet over high heat. Add the bread and cook for 5 minutes, or until brown and crisp. Remove from the pan and set aside.

4 Divide the salad greens among 4 serving plates and add the roasted onions.

5 To make the dressing, whisk the garlic, vinegar, and oil together in a bowl. Stir in the parsley and season with pepper to taste. Drizzle over the salad and onions.

6 Heat the remaining oil in a skillet. Add the cremini and shiitake mushrooms and cook for 2–3 minutes, stirring frequently. Add the oyster mushrooms and cook for an additional 2–3 minutes. Divide the hot mushroom mixture among the 4 plates. Scatter over the pine nuts and croutons and serve.

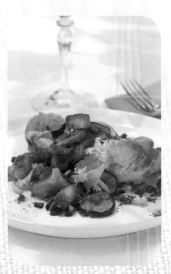

39

SWEET POTATOES

The orange-fleshed sweet potato is high in carotenes and cholesterol-lowering compounds, and is an ideal food for dieters to ward off hunger with.

DID YOU KNOW?

Research has found that sweet potatoes are one of the oldest foods in the world, existing since prehistoric times. They contain naturally occurring substances that can crystallize, and people with kidney or gall bladder problems may be advised not to eat them.

MAJOR NUTRIENTS PER 5½ oz/150 G SWEET POTATO

Kcalories	129
Total fat	Trace
Protein	2.4 g
Carbohydrate	30.2 g
Fiber	4.5 g
Vitamin C	3.6 mg
Vitamin E	0.4 mg
Potassium	506 mg
Calcium	45 mg
Iron	0.9 mg
Magnesium	38 mg
Zinc	0.5 mg
Selenium	0.9 mcg
Beta-carotene	12,760 mcg

Sweet potatoes have a creamy texture and a sweet, slightly spicy flavor. There are two varieties, one with white-cream flesh—also called yams—and the other with orange flesh. The orange variety contains the most nutrients and is the variety referred to here. Sweet potatoes are richer in nutrients than potatoes and lower on the glycemic index, and so are of benefit for diabetics and dieters and for regulating blood sugar levels. They also contain plant sterols and pectin that can help lower "bad" blood cholesterol. They are extremely high in beta-carotene as well as being an excellent source of vitamin E, magnesium, and selenium.

- Carotenes have strong anticancer action.
- Sterols and pectin content help reduce "bad" cholesterol.
- Low glycemic index—good for dieters.
- Antioxidants and vitamin E help improve skin conditions.
- High potassium content helps regulate body fluids and prevent fluid retention.

Practical tips:

Sweet potatoes can be substituted for normal potatoes in many recipes but, unlike potatoes, their skins are often waxed or treated with chemicals and are therefore not always suitable for eating. They can be added to curries, pasta, casseroles, and soup, or roasted, mashed with oil, and baked, halved, and served drizzled with oil. The addition of oil helps carotene absorption.

Sweet potato curry with lentils

SERVES 2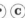

1 tsp canola oil

3½ oz/100 g, peeled weight, sweet potato, cut into bite-size cubes

2¾ oz/75 g, peeled weight, potato, cut into bite-size cubes

1 small onion, finely chopped

1 small garlic clove, finely chopped

1 small fresh green chile, seeded and chopped

½ tsp ground ginger

heaping ¼ cup uncooked green lentils

generous ¼–⅓ cup hot vegetable stock

½ tsp garam masala

1 tbsp low-fat plain yogurt

pepper

Method

1 Heat the oil in a nonstick saucepan with a lid. Add the sweet potato and sauté over medium heat, turning occasionally, for 5 minutes.

2 Meanwhile, place the potato in another saucepan, cover with water, and bring to a boil. Reduce the heat and simmer for 6 minutes, or until almost cooked. Drain and set aside.

3 When the sweet potato cubes are sautéed, remove them with a slotted spoon and add the onion to the pan. Cook for 5 minutes, or until transparent. Add the garlic, chile, and ginger and stir for 1 minute. Return the sweet potato to the pan with the boiled potato and the lentils, half the stock, pepper, and garam masala. Stir well and bring to a simmer. Cover and simmer for 20 minutes, adding a little water if the curry looks too dry. Stir in the yogurt and serve.

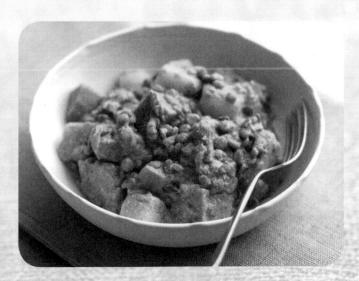

40

ONIONS

The onion is a top health food, containing sulfur compounds that are natural antibiotics offering protection from cancers and heart disease.

Onions are rich in the powerful compound diallyl sulphide, which gives them their strong smell and helps prevent cancer by blocking the effects of carcinogens (cancer-causing particles) in the body. Onions also contain numerous flavonoids, such as quercetin, and these antioxidant compounds help prevent blood clots, and protect against heart disease and cancer. The vegetable also has anti-inflammatory and antibacterial action and can help minimize the nasal congestion of a cold. In addition, onions are very rich in chromium, a trace mineral that helps cells respond to insulin, and are a good source of vitamin C and other trace elements.

- Can help protect against several cancers, including lung cancer.
- Help protect the heart and circulatory system and may increase "good" blood cholesterol.
- Anti-inflammatory, which may help symptoms of arthritis.
- Antibacterial and may help control colds.
- Can help regulate insulin response.

Practical tips:
Stored in an airy, dry, cool place without touching each other, most onions will last for several months, although the vitamin C content will diminish over time. To cook, onions should be gently sautéed in oil to retain maximum nutrients. Mild onions can be thinly sliced and eaten raw.

DID YOU KNOW?
If you cook onions quickly at a high heat, you destroy a large percentage of the beneficial sulfide compounds that they contain.

MAJOR NUTRIENTS PER 5½ oz/150 G ONION

Kcalories	63
Total fat	Trace
Protein	1.4 g
Carbohydrate	15 g
Fiber	2.1 g
Vitamin C	9.6 mg
Folate for	29 mcg
Niacin	1.5 mg
Calcium	33 mg
Potassium	216 mg
Magnesium	28 mg
Selenium	0.8 mcg
Chromium	24 mcg

Roasted red onion soup with cornmeal croutons

SERVES 4

1 lb 12 oz/800 g red onions,
    quartered
1 tbsp olive oil
1 tbsp margarine
generous 1 cup dry white wine
5 cups vegetable stock
1 fresh rosemary sprig, plus extra
    to garnish
1 tsp chopped fresh thyme
1 tsp Dijon mustard
salt and pepper

Croutons

1¼ cups water
2¼ oz/60 g fine instant cornmeal
½ tsp salt
1 tbsp chopped fresh rosemary
olive oil, for brushing

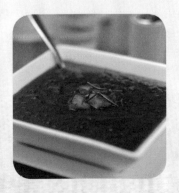

Method

1 Preheat the oven to 400°F/200°C. Place the onions and oil in a roasting pan and toss to coat. Dot with the margarine, season with salt to taste and roast in the preheated oven for 45 minutes, turning occasionally, until very tender and slightly blackened around the edges. Remove from the oven and let cool slightly.

2 Discard the outer layer of each onion segment if crisp, then cut the remainder into thick slices. Place the onions into a large, heavy-bottom saucepan with the wine and bring to a boil. Cook until most of the wine has evaporated and the smell of alcohol has disappeared.

3 Stir in the stock and herbs and cook over medium–low heat for 30–35 minutes, or until reduced and thickened. Stir in the mustard and season with salt and pepper to taste.

4 Meanwhile, to make the cornmeal croutons, heat the water to boiling point in a saucepan. Pour in the cornmeal in a steady stream and cook, stirring continuously with a wooden spoon, for 5 minutes, or until thickened and the mixture starts to come away from the sides of the saucepan. Stir in the salt and rosemary.

5 Cover a cutting board with a sheet of plastic wrap, then, using a palette knife, spread out the cornmeal in an even layer about ½ inch/1 cm thick. Let cool and firm up. Cut into bite-size cubes, brush with oil, and arrange on a baking sheet. Cook in the preheated oven, turning occasionally, for 10–15 minutes, or until crisp and lightly golden brown.

6 Remove and discard the rosemary. Transfer half the soup to a food processor or blender and process until smooth, then return to the saucepan and stir well. Ladle the soup into warmed bowls and serve topped with the cornmeal croutons and rosemary sprigs.

41

BEAN SPROUTS

Bean sprouts are a very low-calorie source of many nutrients, including vitamin C, protein, calcium, and folate.

While you can sprout many types of bean, many of the sprouted seeds available in the stores are from the mung bean. Other sprouts you may find include alfalfa, azuki, lentils, and peas. Bean sprouts are a very low-calorie source of nutrients and thus are very useful for dieters. Dried beans contain no vitamin C, but once they are sprouted by using water, they contain good levels of the vitamin. Bean sprouts are also a good source of protein and calcium, and are rich in folate, the vitamin important for healthy blood and essential for a healthy fetus in pregnant women.

- Low in calories and a rich source of very low-fat protein.
- Good source of vitamin C.
- Very good source of folate.
- Good source of several minerals including iron, magnesium, calcium, and potassium.

Practical tips:
Most beans can be easily sprouted by putting a layer on damp paper towels in a dark place for several days and watering daily. You can also purchase dedicated sprouters. Bean sprouts quickly lose their vitamin C after sprouting, so eat them as soon as possible. They can be used raw in salads and spring rolls, can be stir-fried or lightly steamed, or used as a garnish.

DID YOU KNOW?

Raw sprouts, especially alfalfa sprouts and mung bean sprouts, have a higher than average risk of being contaminated with *E. coli* or salmonella bacteria, which can cause food poisoning. Be sure to wash all sprouts thoroughly before consuming.

MAJOR NUTRIENTS PER 3½ oz/100 g RAW BEAN SPROUTS

Kcalories	30
Total fat	trace
Protein	3 g
Carbohydrate	6 g
Fiber	1.8 g
Vitamin C	13 mg
Folate	61 mcg
Magnesium	21 mg
Potassium	149 mg
Iron	0.9 mg
Calcium	13 mg

Bean sprout salad

SERVES 4

12 oz/350 g bean sprouts
1 small cucumber
1 green bell pepper, seeded
   and cut into matchsticks
1 carrot, peeled and cut into
   matchsticks
2 tomatoes, finely chopped
1 celery stalk, cut into matchsticks
fresh chives, to garnish

Dressing

1 garlic clove, crushed
dash of chili sauce
1 tbsp light soy sauce
1 tsp wine vinegar
1 tbsp sesame oil

Method

1 Blanch the bean sprouts in boiling water for 1 minute. Drain well
  and rinse under cold running water. Drain thoroughly again.
2 Cut the cucumber in half lengthwise. Scoop out the seeds with a
  teaspoon and discard. Cut the flesh into matchsticks and mix with
  the bean sprouts, green bell pepper, carrot, tomatoes, and celery.
3 Mix the garlic, chili sauce, soy sauce, vinegar, and sesame oil
  together in a bowl. Pour the dressing over the vegetables, tossing
  well to coat. Spoon onto 4 serving plates. Garnish with fresh chives
  and serve.

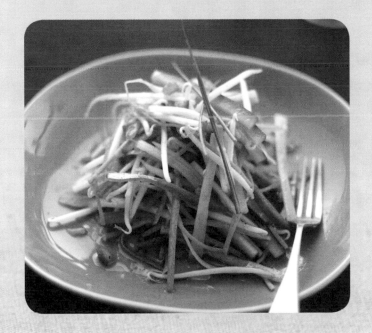

42

LEEKS

As a member of the onion family, leeks have many similar benefits, including an ability to reduce "bad" blood cholesterol and protect against heart disease.

Leeks have a distinct, slightly sweet, onion flavor but are milder than most onions. The long thick stems have a lower white area and dark green tops, which are edible but usually removed because they can be tough and strong-tasting. Leeks have been shown to reduce total "bad" blood cholesterol while raising "good" cholesterol, and so can help to prevent heart and arterial disease. Regular consumption is also linked with a reduction in the risk of prostate, ovarian, and colon cancer. It is the allylic sulfides in the plants that appear to confer the benefits. They are also rich in vitamin C, fiber, vitamin E, folate, and several important minerals.

• Lower total "bad" blood cholesterol and raise "good" cholesterol.
• Anticancer action.
• Mildly diuretic to help prevent fluid retention.
• High in carotenes, including lutein and zeaxanthin, for eye health.

Practical tips:
Wash leeks thoroughly before using—they may contain soil between the tight leaves. The more of the green section of the leek that you use, the more of the beneficial nutrients you will retain. Steam, bake, or stir-fry leeks, rather than boil, to retain their vitamins. The darker green parts take a little longer to cook than the white part so, if chopped, add the green parts to the pan first.

DID YOU KNOW?
In Ancient Greece, leeks were prized for their beneficial effects on the throat. The leek is now the national emblem of Wales, UK.

MAJOR NUTRIENTS PER AVERAGE-SIZED LEEK

Kcalories	61
Total fat	0.3 g
Protein	1.5 g
Carbohydrate	14 g
Fiber	1.8 g
Vitamin C	12 mg
Vitamin E	0.9 mg
Folate	64 mcg
Calcium	59 mg
Iron	2.1 mg
Potassium	180 mg
Magnesium	28 mg
Beta-carotene	1000 mcg
Lutein/Zeaxanthin	1900 mcg

Leek and chicken soup

SERVES 6–8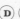

2 tbsp olive oil
2 onions, coarsely chopped
2 carrots, peeled and chopped
5 leeks, 2 coarsely chopped,
   3 thinly sliced
1 chicken, weighing 3 lb/1.3 kg
2 bay leaves
6 prunes, sliced
salt and pepper
fresh parsley sprigs, to garnish

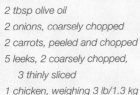

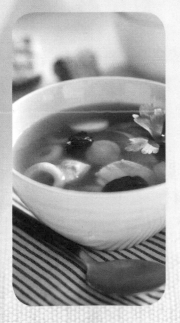

Method

1 Heat the oil in a large saucepan. Add the onions, carrots, and the
2 coarsely chopped leeks and sauté over medium heat for 3–4
minutes, until just golden brown.

2 Wipe the chicken inside and out and remove as much skin and fat
as you can—the breast skin will come away easily with your fingers
and the leg skin can be removed carefully with a small sharp knife
slid between the flesh and skin. Fat clings inside the cavity and on
the underside of the bird.

3 Place the chicken in the saucepan with the cooked vegetables and
add the bay leaves. Pour in enough cold water to just cover and
season well with salt and pepper. Bring to a boil, reduce the heat,
then cover and simmer for 1–1½ hours, skimming off any foam that
rises to the surface with a slotted spoon.

4 Remove the chicken from the stock, remove and discard any
remaining bits of skin, then remove all the meat. Cut the meat into
neat pieces. Strain the stock through a colander, discarding the
vegetables and bay leaves, and return to the rinsed-out saucepan.
Expect to have 5–6 cups of stock. If you have time, it is a good idea
to allow the stock to cool so that the fat may be removed. If not,
blot the fat off the surface with pieces of paper towel.

5 Heat the stock to simmering point. Add the sliced leeks and prunes
and heat for about 1 minute.

6 Return the chicken to the pan and heat through. Ladle the soup
into warmed soup bowls and serve garnished with parsley sprigs.

43 RADICCHIO

The red pigments of radicchio provide anticancer compounds to protect our hearts, and compounds to help prevent blood clots.

Tightly-packed heads of radicchio, sometimes known as Italian chicory, have a strong, slightly bitter flavor that can lift a mixed leaf salad and provide contrasting color. The astringent taste awakens the palate and promotes the secretion of hydrochloric acid, which aids digestion. Radicchio is rich in phenolic compounds, such as quercetin glycosides, which help prevent precancerous substances from causing damage in the body, and anthocyanins, which help protect against both cancer and heart disease. The total phenolic content in red forms of radicchio is about 4–5 times higher than in green varieties. Radicchio also contains good levels of vitamin C, potassium, and folate.

- Acts as a digestive aid.
- Contains high levels of cancer-blocking compounds.
- Protection against heart disease.
- Rich in lutein and zeaxanthin for eye health.

Practical tips:
Look for firm heads with crisp, colorful leaves and no signs of wilting or browning. Store in a plastic bag in the refrigerator for up to five days. Although usually served raw in salads, radicchio heads can be quartered, basted with olive oil, lemon juice, and seasoning, and lightly broiled or baked. It can also be sautéed in oil and drizzled with balsamic vinegar.

DID YOU KNOW?

The two most commonly available types of red radicchio are Verona, with a small, loose head, burgundy leaves, and white ribs, and Treviso, which has a tighter, more tapered head and leaves that are narrower and more pointed.

MAJOR NUTRIENTS PER 1¾ oz/50 G RADICCHIO

Kcalories	12
Total fat	trace
Protein	0.7 g
Carbohydrate	2.2 g
Fiber	0.5 g
Vitamin C	4 mg
Folate	30 mcg
Potassium	151 mg
Calcium	10 m
Selenium	0.5 mg
Lutein/Zeaxanthin	4416 mcg

Red bell pepper and radicchio salad

SERVES 4

2 red bell peppers

1 head radicchio, separated
into leaves

4 cooked whole beets, cut into
matchsticks

12 radishes, sliced

4 scallions, finely chopped

crusty bread, to serve

French dressing

6 tbsp olive oil

1½ tbsp red wine vinegar

1 level tsp superfine sugar

1 level tsp Dijon mustard

salt and pepper

Method

1 Core and seed the bell peppers and cut into rounds.

2 Arrange the radicchio leaves in a salad bowl. Add the bell pepper, beets, radishes, and scallions. Mix all the dressing ingredients together and drizzle over the salad. Serve with bread.

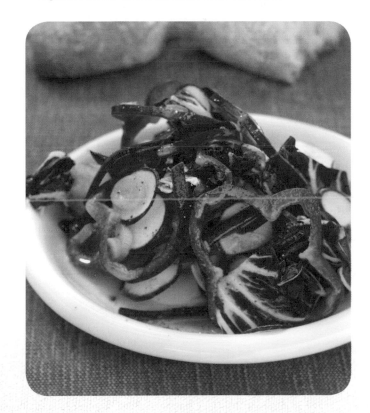

44

ARUGULA

This deep green, peppery salad leaf contains carotenes, which have several cancer-preventing qualities.

Arugula, a member of the brassica family that grows wild across much of Europe, is closely related to the mustard plant. It is a small plant with elongated, serrated leaves. Today, much of the arugula we buy is cultivated but wild arugula leaves contain more of the protective plant chemicals than cultivated hybrids. The leaves are rich in carotenes and are an excellent source of lutein and zeaxanthin for eye health, including cataracts. The indoles contained in arugula and other brassicas are linked with protection from colon cancer. The leaves also supply good amounts of folate—especially important in pregnancy because it helps protect the fetus—and calcium for healthy bones and heart.

- Contains carotenes to protect against cancers.
- Lutein content helps protect eye health, especially in the elderly.
- Contains indoles, linked with a reduction in the risk of colon cancer.
- Good source of calcium for bone protection.

Practical tips:
When buying arugula, the deeper color the leaves, the more carotenes they contain. Arugula can be used in salads or as a garnish. Alternatively, it can be stirred into pasta instead of spinach, made into a pesto, or added to the top of pizza. It doesn't keep fresh for long, so use within one to two days.

DID YOU KNOW?

Arugula grows quickly from seed and is ideal for window boxes or tubs.

MAJOR NUTRIENTS PER ½ oz/15 g ARUGULA

Kcalories	4
Total fat	Trace
Protein	0.4 g
Carbohydrate	0.5 g
Fiber	0.2 g
Vitamin C	2.3 mg
Folate	15 mcg
Potassium	55 mg
Calcium	24 mcg
Beta-carotene	214 mcg
Lutein/Zeaxanthin	533 mcg

Anchovies with celery and arugula

SERVES 4 (D)(P)(C)

2 celery stalks
4 small handfuls of arugula
12–16 brine-cured anchovy fillets,
  halved lengthwise
1½ tbsp extra virgin olive oil
salt and pepper
thick lemon wedges, to serve

Method

1 Quarter the celery stalks lengthwise and slice into 3-inch/7.5-cm sticks. Soak in a bowl of ice-cold water for 30 minutes, or until crisp and slightly curled, then drain and pat dry with paper towels.

2 Place a small pile of arugula in 4 shallow serving bowls. Arrange the celery and anchovy fillets attractively on top. Spoon over a little oil and season with salt and pepper, bearing in mind the saltiness of the anchovies. Serve with thick lemon wedges.

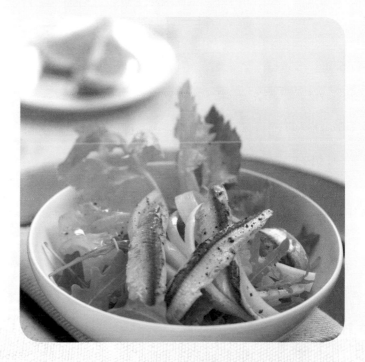

45

WATERCRESS

Peppery watercress leaves are rich in vitamin C and also contain chemicals to help protect us against lung cancer.

Watercress leaves are a powerhouse of nutrients—even if eaten in small quantities—and provide good amounts of vitamins C and K, potassium, and calcium. They are also a great source of carotenes and lutein for eye health. Watercress is rich in a variety of plant chemicals that can help prevent or minimize cancers, including phenylethyl isothiocynate, which can help to block the action of cells that are linked with lung cancer. Watercress is also said to detoxify the liver and cleanse the blood, and the benzyl oils it contains are powerful antibiotics. It can also help improve night blindness and the sun-sensitive condition called porphyria.

- Helps prevent lung and other cancers.
- Detoxifying and blood cleansing.
- Can improve eye health and night blindness.
- High in vitamin K for bone health and healthy blood.

Practical tips:
Buy watercress that has no yellowing or wilting leaves, and store in a plastic bag in the refrigerator or, if bunched, put the bunch in a mug of water up to leaf height. Wash watercress before use and shake to remove excess water. Increase your intake of watercress by using it for a soup with onion and potato. Watercress goes very well with fresh orange segments in a salad.

DID YOU KNOW?
It is best to buy commercially produced watercress rather than searching for wild watercress, as this mainly grows in polluted waters and may carry bacteria.

MAJOR NUTRIENTS PER 1 oz/25 g WATERCRESS

Kcalories	3
Total fat	Trace
Protein	0.6 g
Carbohydrate	0.3 g
Fiber	Trace
Vitamin C	11 mg
Vitamin K	62 mcg
Potassium	83 mg
Calcium	30 mg
Beta-carotene	705 mcg
Lutein/Zeaxanthin	1442 mcg

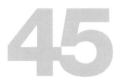

Watercress, zucchini, and mint salad

SERVES 4

2 zucchini, cut into thin sticks

3½ oz/100 g green beans, cut
    into thirds

1 green bell pepper, seeded
    and cut into strips

2 celery stalks, sliced

bunch of watercress

salt and pepper

Dressing

heaping ¾ cup plain yogurt

1 garlic clove, crushed

2 tbsp chopped fresh mint

Method

1 Cook the zucchini sticks and beans in a saucepan of lightly salted,
   boiling water for 7–8 minutes. Drain, rinse under cold running water,
   and drain again. Let cool completely.

2 Mix the zucchini and beans with the bell pepper strips, celery, and
   watercress in a large serving bowl.

3 To make the dressing, mix the yogurt, garlic, and mint together in
   a small bowl. Season with pepper to taste.

4 Spoon the dressing onto the salad and serve immediately.

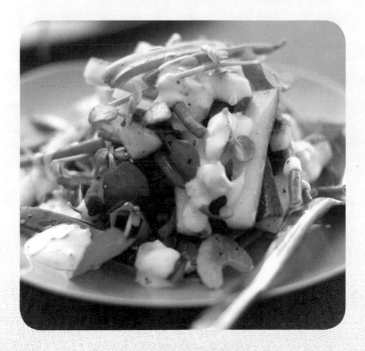

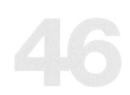

SAVOY CABBAGE

The green leaves of the Savoy contain a range of nutrients and plant chemicals to help fight cancer, and they are also rich in minerals and vitamin C.

Savoy, and other dark green-leaved cabbages are rich in plant chemicals, which may inhibit the growth of cancerous tumors, and which seem to have particular benefit in offering protection from colon, lung, and hormone-based cancers such as breast cancer, probably by increasing the metabolism of estrogen. Cabbage is also very rich in vitamin C, folate, fiber, and minerals, and is a source of B vitamins, vitamin K, iron, and beta-carotene. Its other benefits are that its juice is a traditional remedy for peptic ulcers and its indoles can help lower "bad" cholesterol.

- High in several nutrients, including vitamin C and calcium.
- Proven anticancer and anti-inflammatory effect.
- Helps protect against high "bad" cholesterol and heart disease.
- Can treat peptic ulcers.

Practical tips:
Keep the cabbage stored in the refrigerator in a plastic bag to retain its vitamin C and freshness. To retain most of its nutrients, cook lightly by steaming or stir-frying for a few minutes. To avoid a cabbage odor, don't overcook—cooking with a dash of vinegar also helps.

DID YOU KNOW?

This popular crinkle-leaf cabbage was originally grown in the Savoie, an Alpine region bordering Italy and France, and it is from here that it got its name.

MAJOR NUTRIENTS PER 3½ OZ/100 G SAVOY CABBAGE

Kcalories	27
Total fat	Trace
Protein	2 g
Carbohydrate	6 g
Fiber	3 g
Vitamin C	31 mg
Folate	3 mcg
Potassium	230 mg
Magnesium	28 mg
Calcium	35 mg
Selenium	0.9 mcg
Beta-carotene	600 mcg

Spring stew

SERVES 4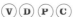

2 tbsp olive oil

4–8 pearl onions, halved

2 celery stalks, sliced

8 oz/225 g baby carrots, scrubbed,
    and halved if large

10½ oz/300 g new potatoes,
    scrubbed and halved,
    or quartered if large

3½–5 cups vegetable stock

14 oz/400 g canned navy beans,
    drained and rinsed

1½–2 tbsp light soy sauce

3 oz/85 g baby corn

¾ cup fresh fava beans

½–1 Savoy cabbage

1½ tbsp cornstarch

2 tbsp cold water

salt and pepper

½–¾ cup freshly grated Parmesan
    cheese or sharp cheddar
    cheese, to serve

Method

1 Heat the oil in a large,
   heavy-bottom saucepan with
   a lid. Add the onions, celery,
   carrots, and potatoes and
   cook, stirring frequently, for 5
   minutes until soft. Add the
   stock, navy beans, and soy
   sauce, then bring to a boil.
   Reduce the heat, cover, and
   simmer for 12 minutes.

2 Add the baby corn and fava
   beans and season with salt
   and pepper to taste. Simmer
   for an additional 3 minutes.

3 Meanwhile, discard the outer
   leaves and hard central core
   from the cabbage and shred
   the leaves. Add to the pan
   and simmer for an additional
   3–5 minutes, or until all the
   vegetables are tender.

4 Mix the cornstarch and water
   together in a small bowl until a
   smooth paste forms, then stir
   into the pan and cook, stirring,
   for 4–6 minutes, or until the
   liquid has thickened. Serve
   with cheese.

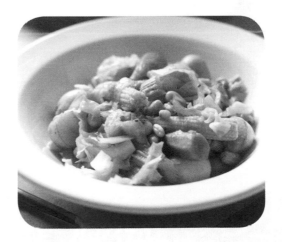

47

CHICORY

Smooth chicory heads are strongly anti-inflammatory, to help minimize the symptoms of arthritis, and their fiber content is a prebiotic for digestive health.

Pale heads of chicory, with their slightly bitter and distinctive flavor, make an ideal addition to a salad. Chicory is blanched during growing by being covered to remove light, as otherwise it would be almost too bitter to eat. It is this bitterness that is linked with the vegetable's beneficial coumarin and lactucin compounds. The anti-inflammatory chemicals they contain can relieve conditions such as gout and arthritis and are said to be sedative. Chicory also contains a special type of fiber, called inulin, which acts as a prebiotic in the digestive system, stimulating the "good" bacteria essential for gut health. It also helps regulate blood sugar levels, boosts the immune system, and can increase "good" cholesterol and reduce "bad" cholesterol.

- Prebiotic for gut health.
- Regulates blood sugar levels.
- Improves blood cholesterol profile.
- Mildly sedative and anti-inflammatory.
- May be mildly laxative.

Practical tips:
Raw chicory is good in salads with orange or pear segments, and is good braised. Chicory heads (chicons) are sensitive to light—keep wrapped in a brown paper bag in the refrigerator. Brush the leaves with lemon juice or vinegar to prevent discoloration.

DID YOU KNOW?

The root of the chicory plant is long and thick, like the taproot of the dandelion. When dried, roasted, and ground, it makes an excellent substitute for coffee.

MAJOR NUTRIENTS PER 1¾ oz/50 g CHICORY

Kcalories	9
Total fat	Trace
Protein	0.5 g
Carbohydrate	2 g
Fiber	1.6 g
Folate	19 mcg
Calcium	10 mg
Potassium	106 mg

Chicory and pear salad

SERVES 4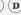

½ cup walnut pieces
2 tbsp maple syrup
2 large pears
juice of ½ lemon
2 heads of chicory, separated
    into leaves
3 oz/85 g bleu cheese

Vinaigrette

4 tbsp olive oil
1 tbsp white wine vinegar
½ level tsp superfine sugar
½ level tsp Dijon mustard
salt and pepper

Method

1 Preheat the broiler to medium–high. Tip the walnuts into a bowl and add the maple syrup. Stir thoroughly to coat the nuts then layer them on a broiler pan covered with foil, leaving any surplus syrup in the bowl. Cook under the preheated broiler for about 2 minutes, or until the nuts are hot and the syrup slightly bubbling. Remove from heat and let cool.

2 Peel, core, and slice the pears lengthwise. Brush each slice with a little lemon juice to prevent discoloration.

3 Mix all the vinaigrette ingredients together in a small bowl.

4 Place the chicory leaves in a bowl and add 4 tablespoons of the vinaigrette. Use your hands to toss together so that the leaves are coated. Add extra dressing, if necessary. Add the pear slices and gently toss again.

5 Divide the salad among 4 serving plates, then crumble the cheese over. Sprinkle the cooled, caramelized walnuts over to serve.

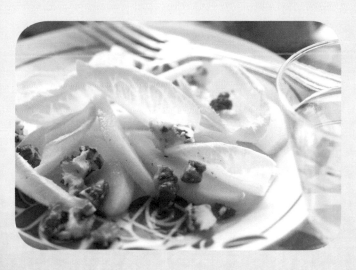

48 SQUASH

Orange-fleshed squash offers protection against lung cancer, and is particularly rich in vitamins C and E.

Squashes are related to pumpkin, cucumber, and melon, and have a lightly nutty flavor that is ideal in both sweet and savory cooking. The orange-fleshed varieties, such as butternut, tend to contain the highest levels of beneficial nutrients. Butternut squash is one of our richest sources of beta-cryptoxanthin, a carotene that is linked with protection from lung cancer. The other carotenes it contains reduce the risk of colon cancer and prostate problems in men. They may also help reduce inflammation associated with conditions such as asthma and arthritis. The vegetable is also a very good source of several vitamins and minerals, including antioxidant vitamins C and E, calcium, iron, and magnesium.

• Contains protective chemicals against lung and colon cancers.
• Anti-inflammatory.
• Rich in a range of vitamins and minerals.
• High fiber source of complex carbohydrates.

Practical tips:
All winter squashes can be stored for up to six months in a cool, dry, dark, airy, frost-free place. To prepare, cut in half with a sharp knife and scoop out the seeds. Squashes can be stuffed and baked, or skinned, sliced, and roasted as an alternative to potatoes. Roast squash makes an excellent soup. The carotenes in squash are better absorbed if you eat them with a little oil.

DID YOU KNOW?

Don't throw away nutritious squash seeds—they can be dried in an oven on a low heat and eaten in the same way as pumpkin seeds.

MAJOR NUTRIENTS PER QUARTER SMALL BUTTERNUT SQUASH

Kcalories	68
Total fat	Trace
Protein	1.5 g
Carbohydrate	17.5 g
Fiber	3 g
Vitamin C	31 mg
Vitamin B3	1.8 mg
Folate	41 mcg
Vitamin E	2.2 mg
Potassium	528 mg
Calcium	72 mg
Iron	1 mg
Magnesium	51 mg
Beta-carotene	6339 mcg
Beta-cryptoxanthin	5207 mcg

Squash, sweet potato, and garlic soup

SERVES 6–8

1 acorn or butternut squash
1 sweet potato, about
*   12 oz/350 g*
4 shallots
2 tbsp olive oil
5–6 garlic cloves, unpeeled
3½ cups chicken stock
heaping ⅓ cup low-fat sour cream
pepper
snipped fresh chives, to garnish

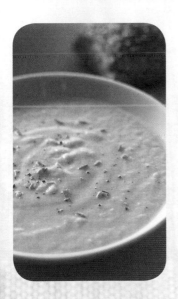

Method

1 Preheat the oven to 375°F/190°C. Cut the squash, sweet potato, and shallots in half lengthwise, through to the stem end. Scoop the seeds out of the squash. Brush the cut sides with the oil.

2 Place the vegetables, cut-side down, in a shallow roasting pan and add the garlic cloves. Roast in the preheated oven for about 40 minutes, until tender and light brown. Cool.

3 When cool, scoop the flesh from the sweet potato and squash halves and place in a saucepan with the shallots. Peel the garlic and add the soft insides to the other vegetables.

4 Add the stock. Bring just to a boil, reduce the heat, and simmer, partially covered, for about 30 minutes, stirring occasionally, until the vegetables are very tender.

5 Let the soup cool slightly, then transfer to a food processor or blender and process until smooth, working in batches, if necessary. (If using a food processor, strain off the cooking liquid and set aside. Process the soup solids with enough cooking liquid to moisten them, then combine with the remaining liquid.)

6 Return the soup to the rinsed-out saucepan. Season with pepper to taste, then simmer for 5–10 minutes, until completely heated through. Ladle into warmed soup bowls and swirl over the sour cream. Garnish with extra pepper and snipped chives and serve.

49 LETTUCE

Mildly sedative, lettuce can help promote sleep. It is also a useful, low-calorie, high-fiber food for dieters.

There are dozens of different types of lettuce available both in the stores and to buy as seed but, when making your choices, for health reasons it makes sense to pick varieties that are either mid- or deep green or with red tinges. These contain more carotenes and vitamin C than the paler lettuces. Romaine lettuce, for example, contains five times as much vitamin C and more beta-carotene than iceberg lettuce. These more colorful heads will contain good amounts of folate, potassium, and iron. Lettuce is high in fiber, very low in calories, and low on the glycemic index.

- Nutritious low-calorie food for dieters.
- High in antioxidant vitamin C and carotenes for disease prevention.
- Mildly sedative.
- High in folate for heart and arterial health.

Practical tips:
Using a clean dish towel or a salad spinner, wash nonorganic lettuces well before use, because sometimes they contain high levels of pesticide residues and bacteria. If a whole lettuce is too much for one meal, pick leaves from the outside rather than cutting it in half, as the cut side will turn brown. Eating lettuce with oil increases absorption of carotenes, but add dressing just before serving so that the leaves do not deteriorate.

DID YOU KNOW?

In most countries, lettuce is usually eaten raw, but in France it is cooked with peas. In China it is often used in stir-fries and other cooked dishes.

MAJOR NUTRIENTS PER 3 oz/80 G LETTUCE

Kcalories	14
Total fat	0.2
Protein	1 g
Carbohydrate	2.6 g
Fiber	1.7 g
Vitamin C	19 mg
Folate	109 mcg
Potassium	198 mg
Calcium	26 mg
Iron	0.8 mg
Beta-carotene	2787 mcg
Lutein/Zeaxanthin	1850 mcg

Green bean and lettuce salad

SERVES 4–6

1 lb/450 g green beans, trimmed

heaping ⅓ cup low-fat mayonnaise

heaping ⅓ cup low-fat plain yogurt

½ tbsp lemon juice, or to taste

½ tsp korma curry paste, or to
    taste

½ tsp ground turmeric

2 hearts of lettuce, leaves
    separated

3 cooked chicken breasts, skinned
    and thinly sliced on the diagonal

salt and pepper

Herb vinaigrette

5 tbsp olive oil

4 tsp white wine vinegar

1 rounded tsp superfine sugar

1 level tsp Dijon mustard

1 rounded tablespoon mixed fresh
    chopped parsley, tarragon,
    and mint

salt and pepper

Method

1 Cook the beans in a large saucepan of lightly salted, boiling water
for 5 minutes, or until tender. Drain them, then immediately plunge
the beans into a large bowl of iced water to stop them cooking, and
let cool completely.

2 Meanwhile, mix the herb vinaigrette ingredients together in a bowl.
When the beans are cool, drain well, and pat dry with paper towels,
then toss them with the vinaigrette and set aside.

3 To make the curry-flavored dressing, mix the mayonnaise and yogurt
together in a bowl until smooth. Add the lemon juice, curry paste,
and turmeric and stir well. Taste and add extra lemon juice or curry
paste, if you like, and a little salt and some pepper to taste. Cover
and chill in the refrigerator until needed.

4 To serve, line a serving platter or individual serving plates with the
lettuce leaves. Place the dressed beans in the center of the platter
or plates. Arrange the chicken slices around the beans, slightly
overlapping, then drizzle the curry-flavored dressing over the
chicken and serve.

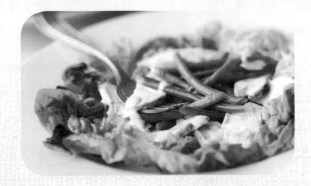

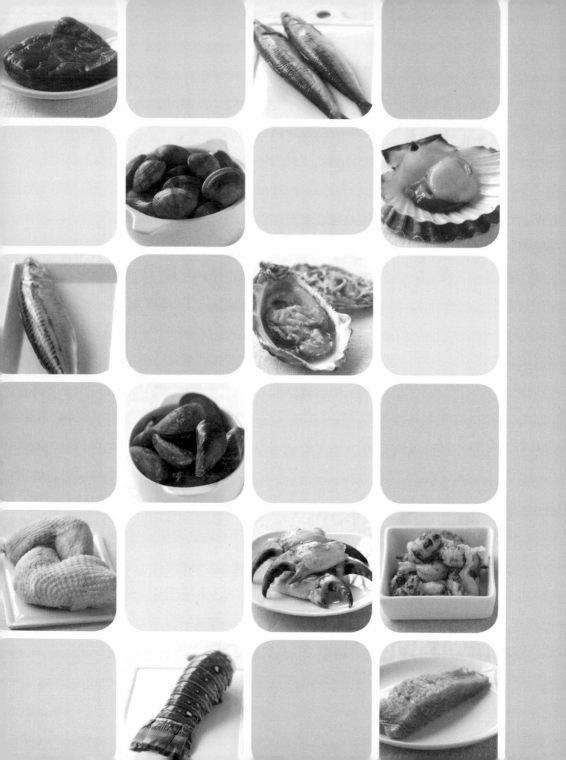

3

CHICKEN, FISH, AND SEAFOOD

Full of omega-3 fats, minerals, and proteins, chicken, fish, and seafood are some of the most important elements to include in a healthy diet. Prepared simply, broiled with delicate flavorings, chicken and fish go well atop any salad or as a meal on their own.

(V) Suitable for vegetarians

(D) Ideal for dieters

(P) Suitable for pregnancy

(C) Suitable for children over 5 years

(Q) Quick to prepare and cook

50 CHICKEN

Grandma was right—scientists have confirmed that chicken soup boosts the immune system and helps fight colds and flu.

Scientists believe that chicken soup relieves the symptoms of colds and flu by stimulating the production of infection-fighting cells. Using chicken bones in the soup greatly boosts the effect. A portion of lean chicken meat contains nearly half of a day's recommended intake of protein for an adult woman, a whole day's intake of niacin (vitamin B3), and makes a large contribution to our intake of minerals such as iron, the antioxidant zinc, and potassium. Chicken is rich in selenium, one of the minerals that is often lacking in our diets, and which has strong anticancer action. Studies also show that organic chicken contains higher levels of omega-3 fats, vitamin E, and other nutrients than nonorganic meat.

- Helps boost immune system and protect against cancer.
- Niacin content helps protect against Alzheimer's disease and cognitive decline.
- B vitamin content helps release energy from our food in the body.
- Vitamin B6 content helps protect arteries from damage from homocysteine, a risk factor for heart disease.

Practical tips:
Fresh chicken should be kept covered in a refrigerator for no more than three days—longer storage increases bacteria count. Wash thoroughly before cooking. Use a separate cutting board for preparing raw chicken and wash hands and utensils carefully.

DID YOU KNOW?

Chicken fat is in its skin. For it to be a low-fat food, you need to remove all the skin before cooking or eating it.

MAJOR NUTRIENTS PER 5½ oz/150 G SKINNED CHICKEN

Kcalories	166
Total fat	4 g
Protein	30.5 g
Niacin	11.8 g
Vitamin B5	1.5 g
Vitamin B6	0.6 mg
Vitamin B12	0.5 mcg
Potassium	356 mg
Selenium	25 mcg
Magnesium	34 mg
Calcium	15 mg
Iron	1.5 mg
Zinc	1.8 mg

Quick chicken laksa

SERVES 4

3 ¾ cups canned low-fat
coconut milk
generous 3 ¾ cup chicken stock
2–3 tbsp laksa paste
3 skinless, boneless chicken
breasts, about 6 oz/175 g each,
sliced into strips
9 oz/250 g cherry tomatoes, halved
9 oz/250 g snow peas,
halved diagonally
7 oz/200 g dried rice noodles
1 bunch fresh cilantro,
coarsely chopped

Method

1 Pour the coconut milk and stock into a saucepan and stir in the laksa paste. Add the chicken strips and simmer for 10–15 minutes over gentle heat, or until the chicken is cooked through.

2 Stir in the tomatoes, snow peas, and noodles. Simmer for an additional 2–3 minutes. Stir in the cilantro and serve immediately.

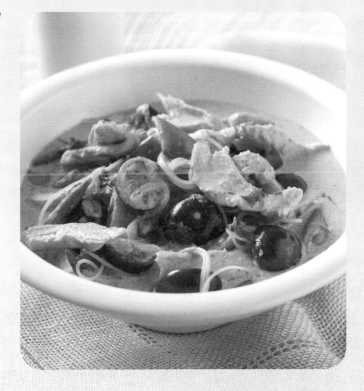

51

TUNA

Fresh tuna is an important source of omega-3 fats and antioxidant minerals for arterial and heart health, and is also rich in vitamin E for healthy skin.

The firm, dense, and meaty, flavorful flesh of fresh or frozen tuna is an ideal choice of fish for nonfish lovers and is quick to cook. It is an excellent source of protein and is especially rich in B vitamins, selenium, and magnesium. A small portion will contain around 20 percent of your daily vitamin E needs. While most types of tuna contain fewer of the essential omega-3 fats than some other oily fishes do, there is still a good content of EPA and DHA fats. DHA is particularly effective in keeping our hearts and brains healthy and in good working order. Just one portion of tuna a week can provide the recommended 1.4 g of these fats a week.

- A good source of omega-3, EPA, and DHA fats, which offer protection against a range of diseases.
- High in protein.
- Rich in selenium and magnesium for heart health.
- Extremely rich in vitamin B12 for healthy blood.

Practical tips:
Fresh fish should be odorless and is best cooked and eaten on the day of purchase. To retain all the health benefits of the omega-3 fats, lightly sear tuna in a pan on both sides and cook for as little time as you can. Tuna steaks can also be sliced and stir-fried for one minute with sliced vegetables—unlike many types of fish, the slices won't disintegrate.

DID YOU KNOW?

Research has found that when tuna is canned (whether in oil, water, brine, or a sauce) it loses most of its beneficial omega-3 fats, so shouldn't count toward your oily fish intake.

MAJOR NUTRIENTS PER 3½ oz/100 G TUNA

Kcalories	144
Total fat	4.9 g
Protein	23 g
EPA	0.4 g
DHA	1.2 g
Niacin	8.3 mg
Vitamin B5	1 mg
Vitamin B6	0.5 mg
Vitamin B12	9.4 mg
Vitamin E	1 mg
Potassium	252 mg
Selenium	36 mcg
Magnesium	50 mg
Iron	1 mg
Zinc	0.6 mg

Seared tuna with white beans and artichokes

SERVES 6

generous ⅓ cup extra virgin olive oil

juice of 1 lemon

½ tsp dried red chili flakes

¼ tsp coarsely ground
 black pepper

4 thin fresh tuna steaks, weighing
 about 1 lb /450 g

1 lb 12 oz/800 g canned cannellini
 beans, well drained and rinsed

1 shallot, finely chopped

1 garlic clove, crushed

2 tsp finely chopped fresh
 rosemary

2 tbsp chopped fresh flat-leaf
 parsley

4 artichokes in oil, drained
 and quartered

4 vine-ripened tomatoes, sliced
 lengthwise into segments

16 black olives, pitted

salt and pepper

lemon wedges, to serve

Method

1 Place 4 tablespoons of the oil in a shallow dish with 3 tablespoons of the lemon juice, the chili flakes, and black pepper. Add the tuna steaks and let marinate at room temperature for 1 hour, turning occasionally.

2 Tip the cannellini beans into a microwavable bowl and heat on medium for 2 minutes. While still warm, toss with 4 tablespoons of the oil, then stir in the shallot, garlic, herbs, and remaining lemon juice. Season with a little salt and plenty of pepper. Let stand for at least 30 minutes to allow all the flavors to develop.

3 Brush a griddle or nonstick skillet with a little of the remaining oil and heat until very hot. Shake off any surplus marinade from the tuna, add to the pan, and sear for 1–2 minutes each side over very high heat. Remove the steaks to a cutting board or plate, reduce the heat to low (or off, for solid stoves), and add the marinade to the pan to cook for 1–2 minutes.

4 Tip the beans into a serving dish. Mix in the artichokes, tomatoes, and olives and any marinade juices from the skillet. Flake the tuna and arrange on top. Garnish with lemon wedges and serve at room temperature.

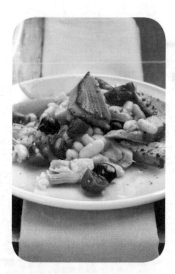

52 SARDINES

Sardines are one of the best sources of omega-3 fats and can protect us against heart and Alzheimer's disease.

Sardines are usually eaten canned, which retains most of the nutrients of fresh sardines, but fresh sardines are a healthy treat. They are one of the richest fish in omega-3 fats, DHA, and EPA. These fatty acids can help prevent or control diseases including arthritis, cardiovascular, and Alzheimer's disease, and an adequate intake can help improve depression and enhance cognitive powers. Sardines are one of the few foods rich in vitamin D, which helps form and protect our bones throughout life. They are also very high in other vitamins and minerals and one portion provides about a third of an adult's daily needs of iron and vitamin E, and a whole day's requirement of vitamin B12 and selenium.

- Excellent source of omega-3 fats for disease prevention.
- Ideal food for long-term brain health and cognitive powers.
- Help lower "bad" blood cholesterol and high blood pressure.
- Regular consumption can provide up to 50 percent reduced risk of stroke.

Practical tips:
Fresh sardines can be cleaned (ask your seller to do this) and then broiled and served with lemon juice and bread, or with broiled tomatoes on whole wheat toast. Sardines can also be filleted for people who don't want to deal with the bones, although the bones are edible and a great source of calcium. Filleted fish can be enhanced with a mustard sauce, which cuts through its richness.

DID YOU KNOW?

Ounce for ounce, sardines provide more protein than steak, more potassium than bananas, and more iron than cooked spinach.

MAJOR NUTRIENTS PER 5 oz/135 g (ABOUT 3) SARDINES

Kcalories	280
Total fat	16 g
Protein	33 g
EPA	1.147 g
DHA	1.550 g
Niacin	7 mg
Vitamin B12	15 mcg
Vitamin	27.7 mg
Vitamin E	2.7 mg
Potassium	536 mg
Selenium	71 mcg
Magnesium	53 mg
Iron	3.9 mg
Zinc	1.8 m

Stuffed sardines

SERVES 6

½ oz/15 g fresh parsley, chopped
4 garlic cloves, finely chopped
12 fresh sardines, cleaned
    and scaled
3 tbsp lemon juice
scant ¾ cup all-purpose flour
1 tsp ground cumin
olive oil, for brushing
salt and pepper

Method

1 Mix the parsley and garlic together in a bowl. Rinse the fish inside and out under cold running water and pat dry with paper towels. Spoon the herb mixture into the fish cavities and pat the remainder all over the outside of the fish. Sprinkle the sardines with lemon juice and transfer to a large, shallow, nonmetallic dish. Cover with plastic wrap and let marinate in the refrigerator for 1 hour.

2 Preheat the broiler. Mix the flour and ground cumin together in a bowl, then season with salt and pepper to taste. Spread out the seasoned flour on a large plate and gently roll the sardines in the flour to coat.

3 Brush the sardines with oil and cook under medium–high heat for 3–4 minutes on each side. Serve immediately.

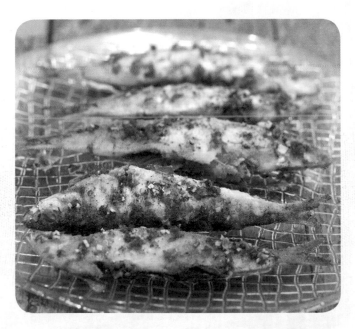

53 MACKEREL

Relatively inexpensive, mackerel is an excellent source of omega-3 fats and is also rich in minerals and vitamin E.

Mackerel is a good choice for everyone seeking their weekly 1–2 portions of oily fish. It is also one of the highest of fish in EPA and DHA—the two special omega-3 fats found in significant amounts almost exclusively in oily fish and fish livers. Multiple scientific papers provide the evidence that increased consumption confers many important, and even vital, health benefits. Numerous trials show that a regular intake of fish oils protects us against heart disease and strokes by reducing inflammation and blood pressure, and improving the blood fat and cholesterol profile.

- Anti-inflammatory that can help symptoms of Crohn's disease, joint pain, and arthritis.
- Can help prevent heart disease and strokes.
- Rich in selenium, magnesium, iron, and potassium, and in vitamins D and E.

Practical tips:
Look for mackerel with firm, shiny bodies and bright eyes. Fresh mackerel won't droop if held horizontally by the head. Oily fish spoils faster than white fish and mackerel is best eaten within 24 hours of purchase. Baking, broiling, barbecuing, or pan-frying are excellent cooking methods and, as it is rich-tasting, instead of creamy sauces, it is best served with sharp or spicy flavors, such as rhubarb sauce, mustard, or horseradish.

DID YOU KNOW?

The Romans used mackerel to make garum, a fermented fish sauce similar to that used in Thai cooking today.

MAJOR NUTRIENTS PER 3½ oz/100 G MACKEREL

Kcalories	207
Total fat	14 g
EPA	0.71 g
DHA	1.1 g
Niacin	9.1 mg
Vitamin B6	0.4 mg
Vitamin B12	8.8 mcg
Vitamin	363 mcg
Vitamin E	1.5 mg
Potassium	317 mg
Selenium	44.5 mcg
Magnesium	77 mg
Iron	1.6 mg
Zinc	0.6 mg

Broiled mackerel

SERVES 4

4 mackerel
2 tbsp olive oil
2 tbsp lemon juice
sea salt and pepper
lemon wedges and cooked
   green beans, to serve

Method

1 Clean the fish and remove the heads. Make diagonal slashes on each side of the flesh. Rub all over with the oil, lemon juice, salt, and pepper, pushing the salt and pepper well into the slashes.

2 Preheat the broiler. Cook under the preheated broiler for 5–6 minutes on each side.

3 Transfer to 4 warmed serving plates and serve with lemon wedges and cooked green beans.

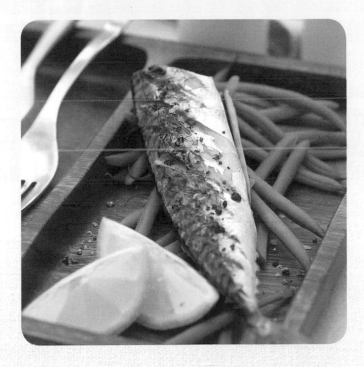

54 SALMON

Salmon is an excellent source of omega-3 fats, of cancer-fighting selenium, and of vitamin B12, which helps protect against heart disease and a form of anemia.

Much of the salmon that we eat today is farmed rather than wild. Although wild salmon tends to contain less fat and a little more of some of the nutrients, the two kinds are broadly comparable. Salmon is our major source of fish oils, which provide protection against heart disease, blood clots, stroke, high blood pressure, high blood cholesterol, Alzheimer's disease, depression, and certain skin conditions. Salmon is also an excellent source of selenium—which protects against cancer—protein, niacin, vitamin B12, magnesium, and vitamin B6.

- Protection against cardiovascular diseases and stroke.
- Helps keep brain healthy and improve insulin resistance.
- May help children's concentration and brain power and protects against childhood asthma.
- Helps keep skin smooth, minimizes sunburn, can help beat eczema, and helps prevent dry eyes.
- Helps minimize joint pain and may protect against cancers.

Practical tips:
For optimum omega-3 content, cook salmon lightly and poach or broil rather than pan-fry. Overcooking can oxidize the essential fats and this means that they are no longer beneficial. Frozen salmon retains the beneficial oils, vitamins, and minerals, while canned salmon loses a proportion of these nutrients.

DID YOU KNOW?
Farmed salmon has been found to contain up to twice the fat of wild salmon—the wild fish is leaner.

MAJOR NUTRIENTS PER 3½ oz/100 g SALMON

Kcalories	183
Total fat	10.8 g
Protein	19.9 g
EPA	0.618 g
DHA	1.293 g
Niacin	7.5 mg
Vitamin B6	0.64 mcg
Vitamin B12	2.8 mcg
Folate	26 mcg
Vitamin E	1.9 mg
Vitamin C	3.9 mg
Potassium	362 mg
Selenium	36.5 mcg
Magnesium	28 mg
Zinc	0.4 mg

Salmon and scallops with cilantro

SERVES 6–8

6 tbsp peanut oil

10 oz/280 g salmon steak,
   skinned and cut into
   1-inch/2.5-cm chunks

8 oz/225 g fresh scallops, shelled

3 carrots, thinly sliced

2 celery stalks, cut into 1-inch/
   2.5-cm pieces

2 yellow bell peppers, thinly sliced

6 oz/175 g oyster mushrooms,
   thinly sliced

1 garlic clove, crushed

6 tbsp chopped fresh cilantro

3 shallots, thinly sliced

juice of 2 limes

1 tsp lime zest

1 tsp dried red chili flakes

3 tbsp dry sherry

3 tbsp soy sauce

cooked noodles, to serve

Method

1 Heat the oil in a large skillet or wok. Add the salmon and scallops and stir-fry over medium heat for 3 minutes. Remove from the skillet and keep warm.

2 Add the carrots, celery, bell peppers, mushrooms, and garlic to the skillet and stir-fry for 3 minutes. Stir in the cilantro and shallots.

3 Stir in the lime juice and zest, dried chili flakes, sherry, and soy sauce, then return the salmon and scallops to the skillet and stir-fry carefully for another minute. Transfer to warmed individual serving plates and serve immediately on a bed of cooked noodles.

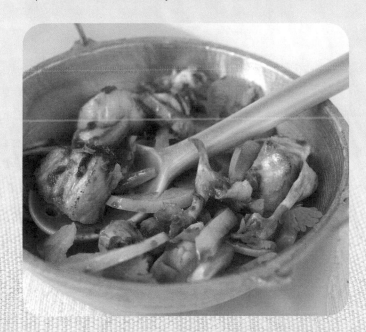

55

CLAMS

Low in fat and high in protein, clams are an ideal food for dieters and they are rich in calcium for a healthy heart and bones.

There are various types of clams available, ranging in size and shape. All edible clams are highly nutritious, being low in fat and high in a wide range of minerals and B vitamins. Clams have a particularly high iron content and just 3½ oz/100 g of shelled clams provide a whole day's intake. Iron carries oxygen from the lungs to all parts of the body and is vital for our immune system, helping to increase resistance to infection and help the healing process. For women who are likely to suffer from anemia due to iron loss during menstruation, eating clams is a great way to replenish iron in the blood.

- High in iron for healthy blood.
- Provide high amounts of calcium for strong bones.
- High in selenium, the anticancer mineral.
- Good source of zinc to boost the immune system and fertility.

Practical tips:
Care should be taken when "shucking" clams (removing them from their shells). The clam should be held in a thick cloth and a proper shucking knife used to pry open the shell. Clams in their shells can be cooked like mussels—in a little liquid over high heat with a lid on. Any that don't open after 3 minutes should be discarded. Clams go well with spaghetti, or can be used in a seafood chowder soup. Clams marry well with garlic, parsley, and tomato.

DID YOU KNOW?

Clams are usually found buried in sand or mud. Although native to both salt and freshwater, saltwater clams are considered to have a superior flavor.

MAJOR NUTRIENTS PER 3½ oz/100 G SHELLED CLAMS

Kcalories	74
Total fat	0.9 g
Protein	12.8 g
Niacin	1.8 g
Vitamin B12	49.4 mcg
Folate	16 mcg
Potassium	314 mg
Selenium	24 mcg
Magnesium	9 mg
Zinc	1.4 mg
Calcium	46 mg
Iron	14 mg

Clams in black bean sauce

SERVES 2

2 lb/900 g small clams

1 tbsp canola oil

1 tsp finely chopped fresh ginger

1 tsp finely chopped garlic

1 tbsp fermented black beans,
rinsed and coarsely chopped

2 tsp Chinese rice wine or
dry sherry

1 tbsp finely chopped
scallion

1 tsp salt (optional)

Method

1 Wash the clams thoroughly, let soak in clean water until you are ready to use them.

2 Heat a wok over high heat for 30 seconds. Add the oil, swirl it around, and heat for 30 seconds. Add the ginger and garlic and stir-fry until fragrant. Add the black beans and cook for 1 minute.

3 Add the clams and rice wine and stir-fry over high heat for 2 minutes to combine all the ingredients, then cover and cook for 3 minutes. Add the scallion and salt, if using, and serve immediately.

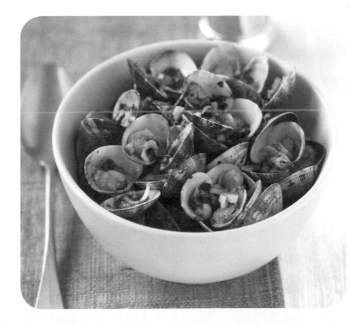

56 SCALLOPS

They may be a luxurious treat but scallops can also help boost your vitamin B12 and magnesium intake to protect the arteries and bones.

Scallops are an excellent source of vitamin B12, which is needed by the body to deactivate homocysteine, a chemical that can damage blood vessel walls. High homocysteine levels are also linked with osteoporosis. A recent study found that osteoporosis occurred more frequently among women whose vitamin B12 status was deficient. A high intake of vitamin B12 has also been shown to be protective against colon cancer. Scallops are also a very good source of magnesium and a regular intake helps build bone, release energy, regulate nerves, and keep the heart healthy. Deficiency can cause abnormal heart rhythms.

- Low in calories and fat so ideal for dieters.
- Rich in magnesium, which has several roles to play in body maintenance.
- A good source of vitamin B12 for arterial and bone health.
- Regular intake may help to protect against colon cancer.

Practical tips:
Fresh scallops should have flesh that is white and firm, have no evidence of browning, and be free of odor. Scallops should only be cooked for a few minutes since exposure to too much heat will cause them to become tough. The sweet flavor of scallops goes well with chile, cilantro, garlic, and parsley.

DID YOU KNOW?
Scallops are rich in tryptophan, an amino acid that helps the production of the mood-enhancing serotonin in our brains and may help cure insomnia.

MAJOR NUTRIENTS PER 3½ oz/100 G SHELLED SCALLOPS

Kcalories	88
Total fat	0.8 g
Protein	16.8 g
Vitamin B12	1.5 g
Folate	16 mcg
Potassium	314 mg
Selenium	22 mcg
Magnesium	56 mg
Zinc	0.95 mg
Calcium	24 mg

Scallops on noodles

SERVES 4

4 oz/115 g dried green tea noodles

2 tbsp low-fat margarine

1 garlic clove, crushed

pinch of paprika

1 tbsp canola oil,
   plus extra for brushing

2 tbsp Thai green curry paste

2 tbsp water

2 tsp light soy sauce

2 scallions, finely shredded, plus
   extra, sliced, to garnish

12 fresh raw scallops, shelled

salt and pepper

Method

1 Cook the noodles in a large saucepan of boiling water for 1½ minutes, or according to the package directions, until tender, then rinse under cold running water and drain well.

2 Meanwhile, melt the margarine in a small saucepan. Add the garlic and cook, stirring, over low heat for 1 minute. Stir in the paprika and set aside.

3 Heat a large wok over high heat for 30 seconds. Add the oil, swirl it around, and heat for 30 seconds. Stir in the curry paste, water, and soy sauce and bring to a boil. Add the cooked noodles and reheat, stirring gently. Stir in the scallions, then remove from the heat and keep warm.

4 Heat a ridged, cast-iron grill pan over high heat and brush lightly with oil. Add the scallops to the pan and cook, brushing with the garlic margarine, for 3 minutes, then turn over and cook for no more than 2 minutes on the other side until just cooked (the center shouldn't be totally opaque if cut open). Season with salt and pepper to taste. Divide the noodles among 4 serving dishes and top with 3 scallops each. Garnish with scallion slices and serve.

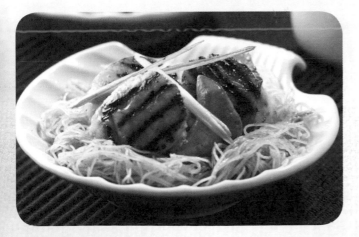

57 OYSTERS

Prized for their nutritional qualities, oysters are rich in zinc, which boosts fertility and skin health, wound healing, and immune-boosting properties.

Although there is little scientific evidence that oysters are an aphrodisiac, they are one of our best sources of zinc and this mineral is strongly linked with fertility and virility. Zinc is also important for skin health, wound healing, and the immune system, and is an antioxidant. Recent research has found that ceramide compounds in oysters inhibit the growth of breast cancer cells. Oysters also contain a reasonable amount of essential omega-3 fats, are rich in selenium for a healthy immune system, and contain easily absorbed iron for energy and healthy blood.

- Excellent source of zinc for fertility and virility.
- Contain compounds and minerals, which can protect against cancers.
- High iron content for energy, resistance to infection, and healthy blood.
- A good source of B vitamins.

Practical tips:
Oysters need to be very fresh and, if eaten raw, they should be alive. It is safest to eat farmed oysters because in recent years wild oysters have been found to contain toxic levels of contaminants. A healthy way to serve fresh oysters is simply topped with chopped shallots, chile, lime juice, and arugula.

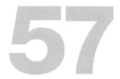

DID YOU KNOW?
Traditionally, an oyster is eaten "all in one go" from the shell, without chewing. You can also cook oysters but some of the beneficial compounds may be lost.

MAJOR NUTRIENTS PER 6 OYSTERS

Kcalories	50
Total fat	1.3 g
Protein	4.4 g
Vitamin B12	13.6 mcg
Folate	15 mcg
Selenium	53.5 mcg
Magnesium	28 mg
Zinc	31.8 mg
Calcium	37 mg
Iron	4.9 mcg

Oysters Rockefeller

MAKES 24

24 large live oysters
rock salt
1 tbsp low-fat margarine
2 tbsp light olive oil
6 scallions, chopped
1 large garlic clove, crushed
3 tbsp finely chopped celery
1½ oz/40 g watercress sprigs
3 oz/85 g young spinach leaves,
    rinsed and any tough
    stems removed
1 tbsp anise-flavored liqueur
4 tbsp fresh breadcrumbs
few drops of hot pepper sauce,
    to taste
pepper
lemon wedges, to serve

Method

1 Preheat the oven to 400°F/200°C. Shuck the oysters, running an oyster knife under each oyster to loosen it from its shell. Pour off the liquor. Arrange a ½–¾-inch/1–2-cm layer of salt in a roasting pan large enough to hold the oysters in a single layer, or use 2 roasting pans. Nestle the oyster shells in the salt so that they remain upright. Cover with a thick, damp dish towel and let chill while you make the topping.

2 If you don't have oyster plates with indentations that hold the shells upright, line 4 plates with a layer of salt deep enough to hold 6 shells upright. Set the plates aside.

3 Melt half the margarine and the oil in a large skillet. Add the scallions, garlic, and celery and cook, stirring frequently, over medium heat for 2–3 minutes, until softened.

4 Stir in the remaining margarine, then add the watercress and spinach and cook, stirring continuously, for 1 minute, or until the leaves wilt. Transfer to a small food processor or blender and add the liqueur, breadcrumbs, hot pepper sauce, and pepper. Process until well blended.

5 Spoon 2–3 teaspoons of the sauce over each oyster. Bake in the preheated oven for 20 minutes. Transfer to the prepared plates and serve with lemon wedges.

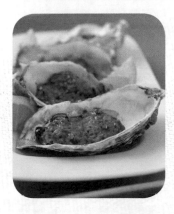

58 MUSSELS

Inexpensive and delicious, mussels are a source of protein, B vitamins for nerve health, and iodine for thyroid function.

MAJOR NUTRIENTS PER 3½ oz/100 G SHELLED MUSSELS

Kcalories	86
Total fat	2.2 g
Protein	11.9 g
EPA	0.41 g
DHA	0.16 g
Vitamin C	8 mg
Niacin	1.6 mcg
Vitamin B12	12 mcg
Folate	42 mg
Vitamin E	0.55 mg
Selenium	44.5 mcg
Magnesium	34 mg
Potassium	320 mg
Zinc	1.6 mg
Calcium	26 mg
Iron	3.9 mg

Mussels are low in saturated fat and high in protein, while also containing some omega-3 essential fats and a wide range of vitamins and many minerals in excellent amounts. They are also low in cholesterol. A portion of mussels will provide around a third of a day's recommended intake of iron for an adult, and about three-quarters of a day's selenium requirement. Mussels are a very good source of B vitamins, providing over 100 percent of daily B12 needs, a quarter of necessary folate, and a useful amount of niacin. Like most shellfish, mussels are also a good source of fluoride for healthy teeth and iodine for healthy thyroid function.

• A low-calorie, low-fat source of good quality protein.
• Contain useful amounts of omega-3 essential fats.
• Rich in iron and selenium.
• Good source of B vitamins.

Practical tips:
Fresh mussels should not smell fishy or of iodine, they should have a slight briny odor. Farmed mussels are considered safer to eat than wild mussels, which can harbor toxins from the sea. Discard any live mussels that don't close tight when tapped and, once cooked, discard any that have failed to open. Mussels go very well with garlic, parsley, and white wine and can be added to fish stews, soups, paella, and shellfish salads.

Mussels with mustard seeds and shallots

SERVES 4

4 lb 8 oz/2 kg live mussels,
  scrubbed and debearded
3 tbsp canola oil
½ tbsp black mustard seeds
8 shallots, chopped
2 garlic cloves, crushed
2 tbsp distilled vinegar
4 small fresh red chiles
1¾ cups low-fat coconut milk
10 fresh or 1 tbsp dried curry
  leaves
½ tsp ground turmeric
¼–½ tsp chili powder
salt

Method

1 Discard any mussels with broken shells or any that refuse to close
   when tapped with a knife.
2 Heat the oil in a large skillet or wok with a lid over medium–high
   heat. Add the mustard seeds and stir them around for about
   1 minute, or until they start to pop.
3 Add the shallots and garlic and cook, stirring frequently, for
   3 minutes, or until they start to brown. Stir in the vinegar, whole
   chiles, coconut milk, curry leaves, turmeric, chili powder, and a
   pinch of salt and bring to a boil, stirring.
4 Reduce the heat to very low. Add the mussels, cover the skillet,
   and leave the mussels to simmer, shaking the pan frequently, for
   3–4 minutes, or until they are all open. Discard any mussels that
   remain closed. Ladle the mussels into 4 deep serving bowls, spoon
   over the broth, and serve.

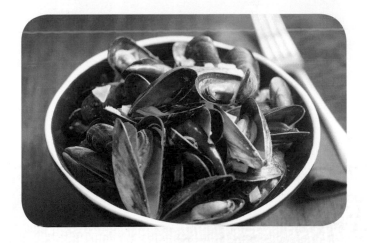

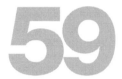

59

CRAB

This low-fat, high-protein shellfish contains l-tyrosine for brain power and high levels of selenium for protection from cancer.

Like mussels, crabs are low in total fat and saturates and rich in minerals. Crabmeat is a good source of l-tyrosine, an amino acid that has been shown to help brain power. It contains as much protein as a similar weight of lean beef and is therefore ideal for vegetarians who eat fish and seafood. A 3½ oz/100 g portion of crab provides over half of a day's recommended intake of selenium, a powerful mineral with anticancer action as well as a quarter of a day's folate. This vitamin helps to protect against birth defects, and is also linked to a reduction in levels of blood homocysteine, which is a contributing factor in heart disease.

- Excellent source of low saturated fat protein, which also contains omega-3 fats.
- Rich in several important minerals.
- Contributes a range of B vitamins in good amounts.
- Very good choice for people watching their weight.

Practical tips:
You can buy live crabs and boil them at home, but many people prefer to buy prepared and dressed crabs, or frozen packages of cooked crabmeat. Unfortunately, canned crab is often high in sodium and has lost much of its omega-3 fats. The white meat is delicately flavored while the brown meat is rich and strong tasting—both are best served simply with lemon and black pepper.

DID YOU KNOW?

There are more than 8,000 species of fresh and saltwater crabs. Every year, over 1 million tons are eaten.

MAJOR NUTRIENTS PER 3½ oz/100 G CRAB MEAT

Kcalories	90
Total fat	4.3 g
Protein	18.5 g
EPA	0.47 g
DHA	0.450 g
Vitamin C	7 mg
Niacin	2.5 mg
Vitamin B12	9 mcg
Folate	44 mcg
Selenium	34.5 mcg
Magnesium	49 mg
Potassium	173 mg
Zinc	2.8 mg
Calcium	26 mg
Iron	2.5 mg

Spicy crab soup

SERVES 4

4 cups chicken stock

2 tomatoes, peeled and
finely chopped

1-inch/2.5-cm piece fresh ginger,
peeled and finely chopped

1 small fresh red chile, seeded and
finely chopped

2 tbsp Chinese rice wine or
dry sherry

1 tbsp rice vinegar

¾ tsp sugar

1 tbsp cornstarch

2 tbsp water

6 oz/175 g white crabmeat,
thawed if frozen or drained
if canned

salt and pepper

2 scallions, shredded, to garnish

Method

1 Pour the stock into a large, heavy-bottom saucepan and add the
tomatoes, ginger, chile, rice wine, vinegar, and sugar. Bring to a boil,
then reduce the heat, cover, and simmer for 10 minutes.

2 Mix the cornstarch and water together in a small bowl until a
smooth paste forms, then stir into the soup. Simmer, stirring
continuously, for 2 minutes, or until slightly thickened.

3 Gently stir in the crabmeat and heat through for 2 minutes. Season
with salt and pepper to taste, then ladle into warmed soup bowls
and serve garnished with scallions.

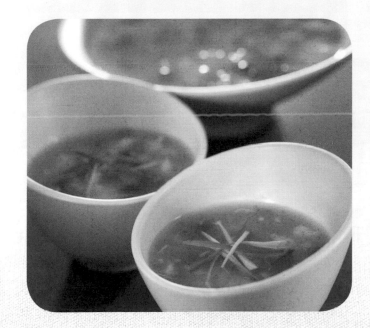

60 CRAYFISH

Low in sodium and rich in vitamin E, crayfish are good for heart health and excellent skin.

Crayfish are freshwater crustaceans—you can find them in some fish markets or as prepared tails in the freezer or chiller cabinets. They have a bright pink appearance, sweet flavor, and make a good substitute for shrimp in recipes. They are much lower in sodium and cholesterol than shrimp and, like most other shellfish, crayfish contain an excellent range of minerals. They are a good source of the antioxidant vitamin E, which is linked with protection from arterial and heart disease, some cancers, and can reduce the pain of arthritis.

• Low in calories and saturated fat.
• Excellent source of vitamin E for health protection.
• Rich in a range of vital minerals.
• Reasonably low in sodium and cholesterol.

Practical tips:
If you buy uncooked crayfish, they should be live. To cook, drop into boiling water for 8–15 minutes, depending on size. Cooked, chilled, or frozen crayfish can be eaten at room temperature or added to stir-fries for the last minute of cooking to heat through. Don't overcook or they will toughen. Try serving cooked crayfish tails on whole wheat toast sprinkled with lemon juice and black pepper, garnished with arugula. Crushed crayfish shells make a good base for a seafood stock or sauce.

DID YOU KNOW?
Crayfish are closely related to lobsters, and have a similar, sweet flavor and nutritional profile.

MAJOR NUTRIENTS PER 3½ oz/100 G CRAYFISH TAILS

Kcalories	77
Total fat	1 g
Protein	16 g
Niacin	2.2 mg
Vitamin B12	2 mcg
Folate	37 mcg
Vitamin E	2.8 mg
Selenium	31.5 mcg
Magnesium	27 mg
Potassium	302 mg
Zinc	1.3 mg
Calcium	27 mg
Iron	0.8 mg

Crayfish in creamy tomato sauce

SERVES 4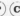

1 tbsp low-fat margarine
1 tbsp olive oil
2 shallots, finely chopped
4 tomatoes, peeled and chopped
2 tbsp tomato paste
pinch of dried oregano
pinch of sugar (optional)
1 lb/450 g peeled crayfish tails
3 tbsp light cream
salt and pepper

To serve
cooked wild rice
handful of arugula
lemon wedges

Method

1 Melt the margarine and oil in a saucepan. Add the shallots and cook over low heat, stirring occasionally, for 5 minutes, until soft. Stir in the tomatoes, tomato paste, and oregano, cover, and simmer gently for 10–15 minutes, until pulpy. Taste, stir in the sugar if the sauce is too sharp, and season with a very little salt and some pepper.

2 Stir in the crayfish tails and heat through gently for 2–3 minutes, stirring occasionally. Stir in the cream and serve immediately on a bed of wild rice, accompanied by arugula and lemon wedges.

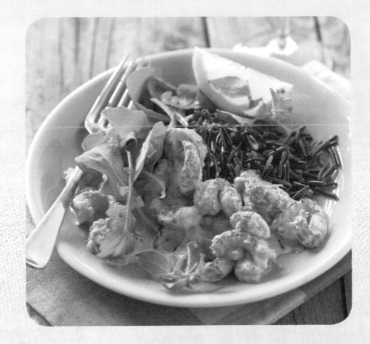

61

LOBSTER

Lowfat lobster flesh is an excellent source of minerals, including zinc, potassium, selenium, and calcium.

For most of us lobster is probably an occasional indulgence rather than an everyday food but, despite its luxurious connection, it is a healthy treat. Lobsters, like crayfish and crabs, are rich in minerals including zinc, potassium, and selenium. They are richer in calcium than many other shellfish and one portion provides about a tenth of a day's recommended intake. Calcium can help to prevent osteoporosis and is important for heart health and muscle function. Lobster is also a very good source of vitamin E, which acts as an antioxidant and helps to keep arteries healthy.

- One lobster portion provides a whole day's selenium intake.
- Very rich source of zinc, the antioxidant mineral that boosts immunity, protects the skin, and is vital for fertility.
- High in pantothenic acid, the B vitamin essential for the conversion of food to energy.

Practical tips:
Fresh lobsters are usually sold live because the meat deteriorates quickly after the lobster is killed. They should be frozen for an hour and then boiled for 15 minutes depending on size. Prepared lobster tails can be bought from the freezer or chiller cabinet of most supermarkets. A large lobster claw yields a lot of meat so don't discard it—simply crush to remove the meat. Cooked lobster tail can be eaten simply as a salad, with lemon juice.

DID YOU KNOW?

Lobsters can live for over 50 years in the wild and are dark blue in appearance. It is only when they are cooked that they become deep pink.

MAJOR NUTRIENTS PER 1 SMALL LOBSTER

Kcalories	135
Total fat	1.35 g
Protein	28 g
Niacin	2 mg
Vitamin B12	1.4 mcg
Pantothenic acid	2.4 mg
Vitamin E	2.2 mg
Selenium	62 mcg
Magnesium	41 mg
Potassium	413 mg
Zinc	4.5 g
Calcium	72 mg
Iron	0.45 mg

Lobster, herb, and saffron mayonnaise salad

SERVES 4

1 lb 10 oz–1 lb 12 oz/750–800 g
 freshly cooked lobster meat,
 cut into bite-size chunks
1 large avocado, peeled, pitted,
 and cut into chunky dice
4 ripe but firm tomatoes
9 oz/250 g mixed herb salad
 greens
1–2 tbsp fruity olive oil
squeeze of lemon juice
salt and pepper

Saffron mayonnaise

pinch of saffron threads
1 egg
1 tsp Dijon mustard
1 tbsp white wine vinegar
pinch of salt
1¼ cups canola oil

Method

1 For the mayonnaise, soak the saffron threads in a little warm water. Meanwhile, put the egg, mustard, vinegar, and salt in a blender and blend to combine. With the motor running, slowly trickle in about one-third of the canola oil. Once the mixture starts to thicken, add the remaining oil more quickly. When all the oil has been incorporated, add the saffron and its soaking water and blend to combine. Add more salt and pepper, to taste, then cover and refrigerate until required.

2 Put the lobster meat and avocado in a bowl. Quarter the tomatoes and remove the seeds. Cut the flesh into fairly chunky dice and add to the bowl. Season the lobster mixture to taste with salt and pepper and gently stir in enough of the mayonnaise to give everything a light coating.

3 Toss the salad greens with the olive oil and lemon juice. To serve, divide between four plates and top with the lobster mixture.

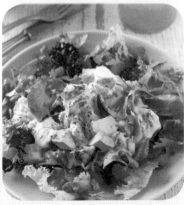

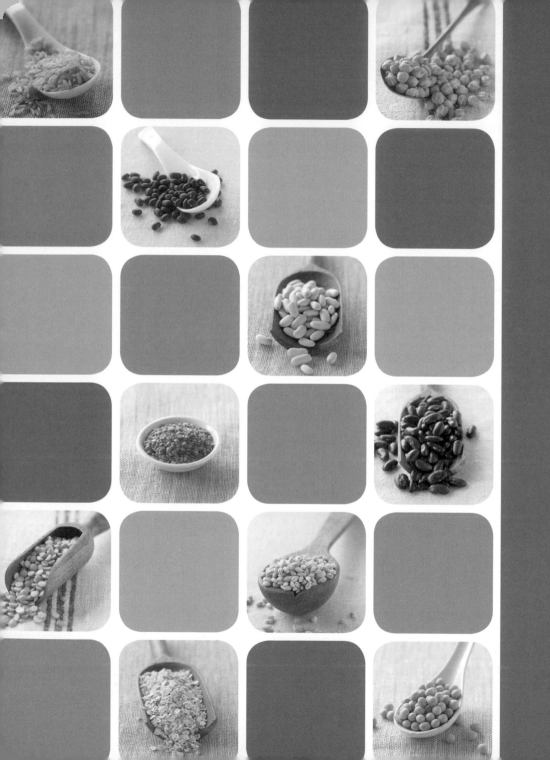

4

GRAINS AND BEANS

There is no better source for fiber or energy-giving carbohydrates than grains and beans. The wide range of diverse textures and flavors allows them to be used in a side dish, as a base for dips, or to enrich sauces or soups.

(V) Suitable for vegetarians
(D) Ideal for dieters
(P) Suitable for pregnancy
(C) Suitable for children over 5 years
(Q) Quick to prepare and cook

62

BROWN RICE

The fiber in brown rice can help to lower blood cholesterol levels and keep blood sugar levels even.

While white rice contains few nutrients other than starch, brown rice has several nutritional benefits. Regular consumption of brown rice and other whole grains has been shown to help prevent heart disease, diabetes, and some cancers. It is a good source of fiber, which can help reduce cholesterol levels in the blood and keep blood sugar levels even. Brown rice also contains some protein, and is a good source of several B vitamins and minerals, particularly selenium and magnesium.

- One of the least allergenic foods.
- A reasonably low glycemic index food that can help control blood sugar levels and may be helpful for diabetics.
- Useful B vitamin content to help convert food into energy and keep the nervous system healthy.
- High selenium content may help protect against cancers, and high magnesium content for a healthy heart.

Practical tips:
Store rice in a cool, dark cupboard and use within a few months. Brown rice tends not to keep as well as white rice as it contains small amounts of fat, which can go rancid over time. The longer you store raw rice, the longer it may take to cook. Leftover cooked rice can be kept for a day or two in a refrigerator if you cool it quickly, but it must be reheated until piping hot before serving.

DID YOU KNOW?
Ninety percent of all rice is still grown and consumed in Asia, where it has been eaten for over 6,000 years.

MAJOR NUTRIENTS PER 2½ oz/60 G RAW BROWN RICE

Kcalories	222
Total fat	1.8 g
Protein	5 g
Carbohydrate	46 g
Fiber	3.6 g
Niacin	3 mg
Vitamin B1	0.2 mg
Vitamin B6	0.3 mg
Selenium	19.6 mcg
Magnesium	86 mg
Iron	0.8 mg
Zinc	1.3 g
Calcium	20 mg

Brown rice vegetable pilaf

SERVES 4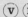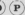

4 tbsp canola oil

1 red onion, finely chopped

2 tender celery stalks, leaves
    included, quartered lengthwise
    and diced

2 carrots, peeled and coarsely
    grated

1 fresh green chile, seeded
    and finely chopped

3 scallions, finely chopped

¼ cup whole almonds, sliced
    lengthwise

1¾ cups cooked brown
    basmati rice

¾ cup cooked split red lentils

¾ cup vegetable stock

5 tbsp fresh orange juice

salt and pepper

fresh celery leaves, to garnish
    (optional)

Method

1 Heat 2 tablespoons of the oil in a high-sided skillet with a lid. Add the
   onion and cook over medium heat for 5 minutes, until softened.

2 Add the celery, carrots, chile, scallions, and almonds and stir-fry
   for 2 minutes, or until the vegetables are tender but still firm to
   the bite, and still brightly colored. Transfer to a bowl and set aside
   until needed.

3 Add the remaining oil to the skillet. Stir in the rice and lentils and
   cook over medium–high heat, stirring, for 1–2 minutes, or until
   heated through. Reduce the heat and stir in the stock and orange
   juice. Season with salt and pepper to taste.

4 Return the vegetables to the skillet. Toss with the rice for a few
   minutes until heated through. Transfer to a warmed serving dish,
   garnish with celery leaves, if using, and serve.

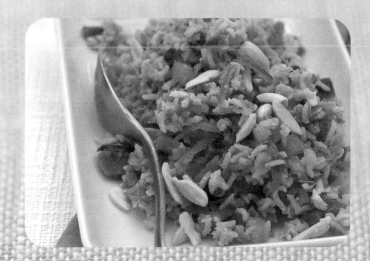

63

CHICKPEAS

Pale, golden chickpeas, sometimes called garbanzo beans, are an excellent, low-cost source of protein, and are rich in fiber, protective plant chemicals, and vitamin E.

Chickpeas are a delicious protein food for vegetarians and a very good source of fiber. Their insoluble fiber, which binds to cholesterol and removes it from the body, not only helps to increase stool bulk and prevent constipation, but also helps prevent digestive disorders such as irritable bowel syndrome and diverticulosis. Its soluble fiber controls and lowers blood cholesterol, and helps prevent strokes and heart disease. Chickpeas are extremely high in folate and this helps lower levels of blood homocysteine, which is a risk factor for cardiovascular disease. They are also rich in magnesium, which helps to relax the arteries and helps protect against heart attacks.

• Very high in folate and magnesium.
• A good source of minerals, including iron, zinc, and calcium.
• High in potassium to help balance body fluids and protect against fluid retention.
• Rich in plant chemicals to fight heart disease and cancer.

Practical tips:
Chickpeas need to be soaked for several hours, then boiled for at least 1½ hours. Chickpeas bought prepared in cans are excellent and still contain the important nutrients. Chickpeas are often eaten in the form of hummus, a Middle Eastern dip, but they can be used to replace meat or poultry in soups, stews, and casseroles.

DID YOU KNOW?

Cooked chickpeas are ground into flour, which is used widely in Middle Eastern and Indian cooking. It is an alternative to wheat flour in many recipes, including batters, breads, and soups.

MAJOR NUTRIENTS PER 2¼ oz/60 g DRIED CHICKPEAS

Kcalories	218
Total fat	3.5 g
Protein	12 g
Carbohydrate	37 g
Fiber	10.3 g
Folate	232 mcg
Magnesium	65 mg
Potassium	393 mg
Zinc	2 g
Calcium	66 mg
Iron	3.9 mg

Chickpea soup

SERVES 6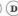

2¼ cups dried chickpeas, soaked
   in cold water overnight

2 tbsp olive oil

1 onion, finely chopped

2 garlic cloves, finely chopped

1 lb/450 g Swiss chard, trimmed
   and finely sliced

2 fresh rosemary sprigs

14 oz/400 g canned
   chopped tomatoes

salt and pepper

slices of toasted bread, to serve

Method

1 Drain the chickpeas and place in a large saucepan. Cover with fresh cold water and bring to a boil, skimming off any foam that rises to the surface with a slotted spoon. Reduce the heat and simmer, uncovered, for 1–1¼ hours, until tender, topping off with water, if necessary.

2 Drain the chickpeas, reserving the cooking water. Season the chickpeas well with salt and pepper. Place two-thirds in a food processor or blender with some of the reserved cooking water and process until smooth, adding more of the cooking water, if necessary, to achieve a soup consistency. Return to the saucepan.

3 Heat the oil in a medium saucepan. Add the onion and garlic and cook over medium heat, stirring, for 3–4 minutes, until the onion is soft. Add the Swiss chard and rosemary and cook for 3–4 minutes. Add the tomatoes and the remaining chickpeas and cook for an additional 5 minutes, or until the tomatoes have broken down to an almost smooth sauce. Remove the rosemary sprigs.

4 Add the Swiss chard and tomato mixture to the chickpea puree and simmer for 2–3 minutes. Taste and adjust the seasoning, if necessary. Ladle into warmed soup bowls and serve with slices of toasted bread.

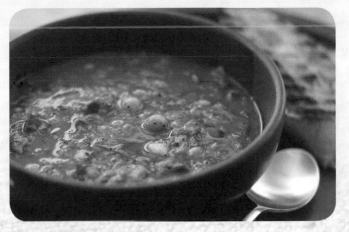

64 BLACK BEANS

Shiny, oval black beans are an ideal and inexpensive addition to the diet, being rich in nutrients and cholesterol-lowering fibers, and very low in fat and saturates.

Black beans are a delicious addition to the diet. Nutritionally, they are high in the indigestible portion of the plant known as insoluble fiber, which can reduce cholesterol. Their extremely high magnesium content means that they are an excellent food for people at risk of developing or suffering from heart disease—an optimum intake of magnesium is linked with a reduced risk of various heart problems. Black beans are also rich in antioxidant compounds called anthocyanins, flavonoids that can help prevent cancer and blood clots. The darker the bean's seed coat, the higher its level of antioxidant activity. In addition, black beans are an excellent source of minerals and folate.

- High fiber food to help beat some cancers and reduce cholesterol.
- Rich in anthocyanins to block cancer cells.
- Contain folate for healthy blood and development.
- A very good source of vegetable protein.

Practical tips:
Buy the beans dried for long storage or ready cooked in cans. Be sure to rinse canned beans packed in brine well before use. Presoaking beans reduces the raffinose-type oligosaccharides contained in them, which are sugars associated with flatulence. Black beans can be used in a range of dishes, from soups and stews to rice dishes and crêpe fillings.

DID YOU KNOW?

Black beans were native to South America but since the 15th century, when they were introduced into Europe by Spanish explorers, they have been popular throughout Europe, Africa, and Asia as well as the United States.

MAJOR NUTRIENTS PER 2¼ oz/60 G DRIED BLACK BEANS

Kcalories	205
Total fat	0.8 g
Protein	13.7 g
Carbohydrate	36.7 g
Fiber	13.5 g
Folate	231 mcg
Vitamin B1	0.4 mg
Magnesium	109 mg
Potassium	550 mg
Zinc	1.7 g
Calcium	42 mg

Black bean sauce

MAKES ABOUT ⅔ CUP

1 tbsp peanut oil

2 tbsp fermented black beans, finely chopped

1 garlic clove, chopped

1 tbsp grated fresh ginger

1 shallot, chopped

2 scallions, finely chopped

2 small fresh green chiles, seeded and chopped

1 tbsp light soy sauce

1 tbsp strained freshly squeezed lemon juice

⅔ cup vegetable stock

1–2 tsp superfine sugar, or to taste

salt and pepper

Method

1 Heat a wok over high heat for 30 seconds. Add the oil, swirl it around to coat the bottom, and heat for 30 seconds. Add the black beans, garlic, ginger, and shallot and stir-fry for 2 minutes.

2 Add the scallions and chiles and stir-fry for 3 minutes. Add the soy sauce and lemon juice and simmer for 2 minutes. Add the stock and sugar with salt and pepper to taste and simmer for an additional 2 minutes. Transfer to a serving bowl and serve as required.

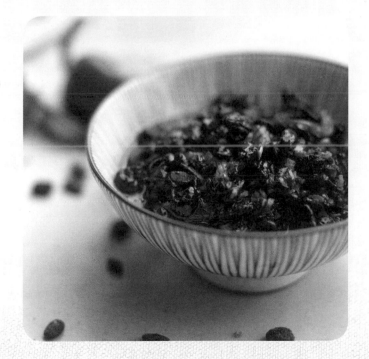

65

NAVY BEANS

High-protein navy beans are often the contents of canned baked beans and are also very high in fiber, minerals, and B vitamins.

Navy beans are a very high fiber food. Their soluble fiber helps to lower cholesterol and prevent blood sugar levels from rising too rapidly after a meal, making these beans a good choice for dieters as well as people with diabetes, insulin resistance, and hypoglycemia. Their insoluble fiber helps to prevent constipation and reduce the severity and symptoms of digestive disorders such as irritable bowel syndrome and diverticulosis. Navy beans are also a good source of protein and one of the best beans for supplying calcium. One portion provides a seventh of a day's recommended intake. They are also very rich in magnesium, potassium, iron, zinc, and are a very good source of B vitamins and folate.

- Rich in soluble fiber to help lower blood cholesterol and protect from cardiovascular disease.
- Insoluble fiber helps the digestive system and bowels.
- A good source of calcium for a healthy heart and strong bones.
- Rich in antioxidant minerals such as zinc to help prevent disease.

Practical tips:
To prepare, soak the beans overnight, then replace the water and boil rapidly for 10 minutes before simmering for about 1½ hours, until tender. Do not add salt to beans before they are cooked, as the salt will make them tough. Cooked beans can be pureed with olive oil, salt, and pepper to make an alternative to mashed potato.

DID YOU KNOW?
Early in the 20th century navy beans were so called because they were a staple food for the US Navy.

MAJOR NUTRIENTS PER 2¼ oz/60 g DRIED NAVY BEANS

Kcalories	200
Total fat	12 g
Protein	0.9 g
Carbohydrate	37.8 g
Fiber	15 g
Folate	203 mcg
Vitamin B1	0.35 mga
Niacin	0.95 mg
Magnesium	77 mg
Potassium	564 mg
Zinc	1.5 g
Calcium	100 mg
Iron	3.4 mg

Navy and green bean salad

SERVES 4

½ cup navy beans, soaked in cold
    water overnight
8 oz/225 g green beans, trimmed
¼ red onion, thinly sliced
12 black olives, pitted
1 tbsp snipped chives

Dressing

½ tbsp lemon juice
½ tsp Dijon mustard
6 tbsp extra virgin olive oil
salt and pepper

Method

1. Drain the navy beans and place in a saucepan. Cover with fresh water and bring to a boil. Boil rapidly for 15 minutes, then reduce the heat slightly and cook for 30 minutes, or until tender but not disintegrating. Add salt in the last 5 minutes of cooking. Drain and set aside.

2. Meanwhile, cook the green beans in a large saucepan of boiling water for 4 minutes, or until just tender but still brightly colored and crunchy. Drain and set aside.

3. Whisk the lemon juice, mustard, oil, and salt and pepper to taste, together in a bowl, then let stand.

4. While both types of bean are still slightly warm, tip them into a shallow serving dish or arrange on 4 serving plates. Scatter over the onion slices, olives, and chives.

5. Whisk the dressing again and spoon over the salad. Serve at room temperature.

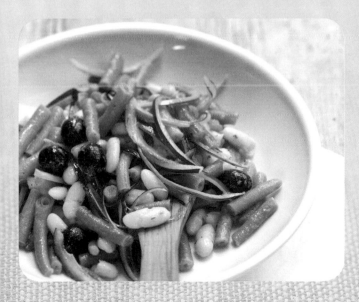

66 KIDNEY BEANS

Iron-rich kidney beans are an excellent source of good-quality protein, zinc, and fiber, and contain compounds to help prevent blood clots.

Kidney beans are invaluable for vegetarians as they are high in good-quality protein and minerals. An average portion of kidney beans contains at least a quarter of our day's iron needs to help prevent anemia and increase energy levels, while their good zinc content helps boost the immune system and maintain fertility. The high degree of insoluble fiber in kidney beans helps prevent colon cancer, while for diabetics and people with insulin resistance, the total fiber content helps regulate blood sugar levels.

- Excellent source of protein, iron, and calcium for vegetarians.
- Very high fiber content helps regulate release of insulin and helps to prevent hunger—a good choice for dieters.
- Protects against colon cancer.
- Extremely high in potassium, which can minimize fluid retention and may help control high blood pressure.

Practical tips:
There is little nutritional difference between dried cooked kidney beans and canned kidney beans so, if you are short of time, use the canned variety. Red kidney beans are often added to meat dishes such as chile con carne, or used in three bean salad and, when mashed with oil and lemon juice, make a good sandwich filling or dip.

DID YOU KNOW?

Raw kidney beans can contain high levels of potentially toxic substances, which can cause an upset stomach, vomiting, and diarrhea. In order to remove this risk, the beans must be rapidly boiled for at least 10 minutes before cooking.

MAJOR NUTRIENTS PER 2¼ oz/60 g DRIED RED KIDNEY BEANS

Kcalories	200
Total fat	0.8 g
Protein	13.7 g
Carbohydrate	36 g
Fiber	10 g
Folate	205 mcg
Vitamin B1	0.25 mg
Niacin	0.9 mg
Magnesium	66 mg
Potassium	640 mg
Zinc	1.6 g
Calcium	55 mg
Iron	3.5 mg

Mushroom and kidney bean chile

SERVES 6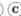

4 tbsp olive oil

8 oz/225 g small button mushrooms

1 large onion, chopped

1 garlic clove, chopped

1 green bell pepper, seeded and cut into strips

1 tsp each paprika, ground coriander, and ground cumin

¼–½ tsp chili powder

14 oz/400 g canned chopped tomatoes

⅔ cup vegetable stock

1 tbsp tomato paste

14 oz/400 g canned red kidney beans, drained and rinsed

salt and pepper

2 tbsp chopped fresh cilantro, to garnish

cooked rice and low-fat sour cream, to serve

Method

1 Heat 1 tablespoon of the oil in a large skillet. Add the mushrooms and stir-fry until golden. Remove them with a slotted spoon and set aside until needed.

2 Add the remaining oil to the skillet. Add the onion, garlic, and green bell pepper and stir-fry for 5 minutes. Stir in the paprika, coriander, cumin, and chili powder and cook for an additional 1 minute.

3 Add the tomatoes, stock, and tomato paste, stir well, then cover and cook for 20 minutes.

4 Add the reserved mushrooms and kidney beans and cook, covered, for an additional 20 minutes. Season with salt and pepper to taste. Garnish with the cilantro and serve with cooked rice and sour cream.

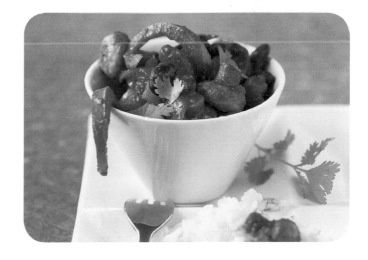

67

LENTILS

Small, lens-shaped dried lentils are one of the beans richest in cancer-blocking fibers called isoflavones and lignan, and are low in fat and saturates.

Lentils come in a variety of colors and include green, brown, and red. The green and brown tend to contain the highest levels of nutrients and fiber. Lentils are a very rich source of fiber, both insoluble and soluble, which helps protect us against cancer and cardiovascular disease. They also contain plant chemicals called isoflavones, which may offer protection from cancer and coronary heart disease, and lignan, which has a mild estrogen-like effect that may lower the risk of cancer, minimize premenstrual syndrome, and protect against osteoporosis. Lentils are also rich in B vitamins, folate, and all major minerals, particularly iron and zinc.

- Rich in fiber for protection from cardiovascular disease and cancers.
- High iron content for healthy blood and energy levels.
- Contain plant chemicals to help premenstrual syndrome and bone health.
- High zinc content to boost the immune system.

Practical tips:
Lentils are one of the few beans that don't need soaking before cooking. They are also quick to cook by simmering in water for about 30 minutes. Dried lentils cooked in stock with carrots, celery, and onion makes a quick soup. Canned lentils contain almost as many nutrients as dried ones.

DID YOU KNOW?

Lentils are thought to be one of the earliest foods to have been cultivated, with 8,000-year-old seeds found at sites in the Middle East.

MAJOR NUTRIENTS PER 2¼ oz/60 G DRIED GREEN OR BROWN LENTILS

Kcalories	212
Total fat	0.6 g
Protein	15.5 g
Carbohydrate	36 g
Fiber	18 g
Folate	287 mcg
Vitamin B1	0.5 mg
Niacin	1.6 mg
Vitamin B6	0.3 mg
Magnesium	73 mg
Potassium	573 mg
Zinc	2.9 g
Calcium	34 mg
Iron	4.5 mg

Mixed lentils with five-spice seasoning

SERVES 4

¾ cup red split lentils

¾ cup skinless split mung beans

3½ cups hot water

1 tsp ground turmeric

1 tsp salt, or to taste

1 tbsp lemon juice

2 tbsp olive oil

¼ tsp black mustard seeds

¼ tsp cumin seeds

¼ tsp nigella seeds

¼ tsp fennel seeds

4–5 fenugreek seeds

2–3 dried red chiles

1 small tomato, seeded and cut into strips and fresh cilantro sprigs, to garnish

flat bread, to serve

Method

1 Mix both types of lentils together and rinse under cold running water until the water runs clear. Place the lentils in a saucepan with the hot water and bring to a boil, then reduce the heat slightly. Let it boil for 5–6 minutes, and when the foam subsides, add the turmeric, reduce the heat to low, cover, and cook for 20 minutes. Add the salt and lemon juice and beat the lentils with a wire beater. Add a little more hot water if the lentils are too thick.

2 Heat the oil in a small saucepan over medium heat. When hot, but not smoking, add the mustard seeds. As soon as they begin to pop, reduce the heat to low and add the cumin seeds, nigella seeds, fennel seeds, fenugreek seeds, and dried chiles. Let the spices sizzle until the seeds begin to pop and the chiles have blackened.

3 Pour the contents of the saucepan over the lentils, scraping off every bit from the saucepan. Transfer to a serving dish and garnish with tomato strips and cilantro sprigs. Serve with flat bread.

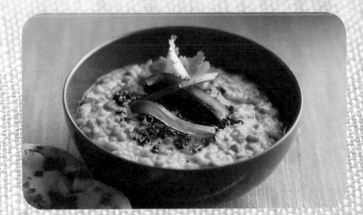

68

SPLIT PEAS

Small yellow or green split peas are very rich in cholesterol-lowering soluble fiber, and are a source of daidzein for protecting against breast cancer.

MAJOR NUTRIENTS PER 2¼ oz/60 g DRIED SPLIT PEAS

Kcalories	205
Total fat	0.7 g
Protein	14.5 g
Carbohydrate	36 g
Fiber	15 g
Folate	164 mcg
Vitamin B1	0.4 mg
Niacin	1.7 mg
Magnesium	69 mg
Potassium	589 mg
Zinc	1.8 g
Calcium	33 mg
Iron	2.6 mg
Beta-carotene	53 mcg

Dried split peas, like other legumes, are rich in soluble fiber. This forms a gel-like substance in the digestive tract that binds cholesterol-containing bile and carries it out of the body. Split peas also contain an isoflavone, called daidzein, which acts like weak estrogen in the body. The consumption of this isoflavone has been linked to a reduced risk of certain health conditions, including breast and prostate cancer. Split peas are particularly rich in potassium, the mineral that can help lower blood pressure, control fluid retention, and may help limit the growth of potentially damaging plaques in the blood vessels.

• Rich in soluble fiber to help lower "bad" blood cholesterol.
• A source of daidzein, which may reduce risk of hormone-related cancers.
• Very high in potassium for heart health.
• Excellent source of vegetable protein.

Practical tips:
Like lentils, split peas don't need to be soaked before cooking and can be simply cooked in simmering water for about 30 minutes. Cooked split peas can be pureed and served as a healthier alternative to potatoes. They can also be pureed with oil and spices to make a dip.

Split pea and ham soup

SERVES 6–8

2½ cups split green peas

1 tbsp olive oil

1 large onion, finely chopped

1 large carrot, peeled and finely
  chopped

1 celery stalk, finely chopped

4 cups chicken or vegetable stock

4 cups water

8 oz/225 g lean unsmoked ham,
  finely diced

¼ tsp dried thyme

¼ tsp dried marjoram

1 bay leaf

salt and pepper

Method

1 Rinse the peas under cold running water. Place them in a saucepan
   and cover generously with water. Bring to a boil and boil for
   3 minutes, skimming off any foam that rises to the surface with a
   slotted spoon. Drain and set aside.

2 Heat the oil in a large saucepan. Add the onion and cook over
   medium heat for 3–4 minutes, until just softened.

3 Add the carrot and celery and cook for 2 minutes. Add the peas,
   pour over the stock and water, and stir to combine. Bring just to a
   boil and stir the ham into the soup.

4 Add the thyme, marjoram, and bay leaf to the pan. Reduce the heat,
   cover, and cook gently for 1–1½ hours, until everything is very soft.
   Remove the bay leaf. Taste and adjust the seasoning, if necessary.
   Ladle into warmed soup bowls and serve.

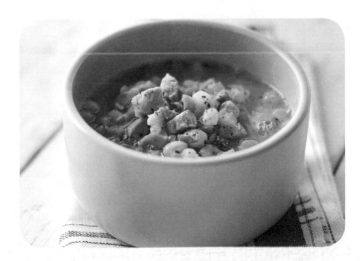

WHOLE GRAIN BARLEY

This extremely nutritious starchy grain contains soluble fiber that helps to lower "bad" blood cholesterol and protect us from hormonal cancers and heart disease.

Whole grain barley is a grain with a rich, slightly nutty flavor and a chewy texture. Most barley that is sold is pearl barley, which has had almost all of the nutrients and fiber removed by processing, whereas whole grain or hulled barley, has had minimal processing and is therefore a good source of nutrients. These include a very high level of fiber, including soluble fiber, and a fiber-like compound called lignan, which may protect against breast and other hormone-dependent cancers as well as heart disease. Unusually for a grain, barley contains lutein and zeaxanthin, which help to protect eyesight and eye health.

- Whole grain that protects against cancers and heart disease.
- A good source of minerals and B vitamins.
- High in fiber to keep the colon healthy and soluble fiber to lower blood cholesterol.
- Helps to keep eyes healthy.

Practical tips:
Whole grain barley needs up to two hours of simmering in water, but presoaking it for several hours will shorten the cooking time. Add it to soups and casseroles for extra nutrition and fiber. The fats in barley can make it go rancid after a short time, especially if kept in warm, light conditions so store in a cool, dry, dark place in an airtight container and use within two to three months.

DID YOU KNOW?

Barley water, made by steeping the grains in water, has long been considered a health drink for its diuretic and kidney-supporting effect.

MAJOR NUTRIENTS PER 2¼ oz/60 G RAW WHOLE GRAIN BARLEY

Kcalories	212
Total fat	1.4 g
Protein	7.5 g
Carbohydrate	44 g
Fiber	10.4 g
Vitamin B1	0.4 mg
Niacin	2.8 mg
Selenium	22.5 mcg
Magnesium	80 mg
Potassium	271 mg
Zinc	1.7 g
Calcium	20 mg
Iron	2.2 mg
Lutein/Zeaxanthin	96 mcg

Hearty barley vegetable soup

SERVES 4–6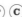

2 tbsp canola oil

1 onion, finely chopped

1 celery stalk, finely chopped

1 garlic clove, crushed

6 cups vegetable stock or water

heaping ⅓ cup whole grain
    barley, rinsed

1 bouquet garni, made with 1 bay
    leaf, fresh thyme sprigs, and
    fresh parsley sprigs

2 carrots, peeled and diced

14 oz/400 g canned chopped
    tomatoes

pinch of sugar

½ head Savoy cabbage, cored
    and shredded

salt and pepper

2 tbsp chopped fresh parsley,
    to garnish

chunky whole wheat bread,
    to serve

Method

1 Heat the oil in a large saucepan. Add the onion, celery, and garlic and cook over medium heat for 5–7 minutes, until softened.

2 Pour in the stock and bring to a boil, skimming off any foam that rises to the surface with a slotted spoon. Add the barley and bouquet garni, reduce the heat to low, cover, and simmer for 30 minutes–1 hour until the grains are just beginning to soften.

3 Add the carrots, tomatoes with their can juices, and the sugar to the pan. Bring the liquid back to a boil, then reduce the heat to low, cover, and simmer for an additional 30 minutes, or until the barley and carrots are tender.

4 Just before serving, remove the bouquet garni, stir in the cabbage, and season with salt and pepper to taste. Continue simmering until the cabbage wilts, then ladle into warmed soup bowls and garnish with parsley. Serve with whole wheat bread.

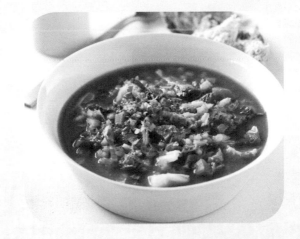

70

OATS

Economical oats are high in soluble fiber and a source of healthy fats. They can keep hunger at bay, lower "bad" cholesterol, and keep blood sugar levels even.

Oats have several health-giving properties. They are rich in the soluble fiber beta-glucan and have been proven to help lower "bad" cholesterol, boost "good" cholesterol, maintain a healthy circulatory system, and help prevent heart attacks. Oats also contain a range of antioxidants and plant chemicals to help keep heart and arteries healthy, such as avenanthramides (a phytoalexin plant chemical with antibiotic properties), saponins, and vitamin E. They also contain polyphenols, plant compounds that can suppress tumor growth. They are also relatively low on the glycemic index, which means they are particularly suitable for dieters, people with insulin resistance, and diabetics.

- One of the best grains to keep the heart and arteries healthy.
- Contain plant chemicals to help reduce the risk of cancers.
- Lower on the glycemic index than many cereals.
- A good source of a wide range of vitamins and minerals, including B vitamins, vitamin E, magnesium, calcium, and iron.

Practical tips:
The fat content of oats means that they don't store well for long, so keep them in an airtight container in a cool, dry, dark place and use within 2–3 weeks. Use oat flakes to make your own homemade muesli. Oat flakes can be used for making cookies and crumble toppings, and oat flour can replace wheat flour.

DID YOU KNOW?

Although oats do contain small amounts of gluten, people with gluten intolerance (celiac disease) often find they can tolerate oats in their diet, especially if limited to no more than ⅔ cup a day. Celiac sufferers should check with their doctor before eating oats.

MAJOR NUTRIENTS PER 2¼ oz/60 G OATS

Kcalories	233
Total fat	4 g
Protein	10 g
Carbohydrate	40 g
Fiber	6.4 g
Folate	34 mcg
Vitamin B1	0.5 mg
Niacin	0.6 mg
Vitamin E	1.5 mg
Magnesium	106 mg
Potassium	257 mg
Zinc	2.4 mg
Calcium	32 mg
Iron	2.8 mg

Oat bars

MAKES 16

1½ sticks low-fat margarine, plus
   extra for greasing
3 tbsp honey
¾ cup raw brown sugar
scant ½ cup smooth peanut butter
3 cups rolled oats
heaping ¼ cup chopped plumped
   dried apricots
2 tbsp sunflower seeds
2 tbsp sesame seeds

Method

1 Preheat the oven to 350°F/180°C. Grease and line a 8½-inch/
   22-cm square baking pan.

2 Melt the margarine, honey, and sugar in a saucepan over low heat.
   When the sugar has melted, add the peanut butter and stir until
   everything is well combined. Add all the remaining ingredients and
   mix well.

3 Press the mixture into the prepared pan and bake in the preheated
   oven for 20 minutes. Remove from the oven and let cool in the pan,
   then cut into 16 squares and serve.

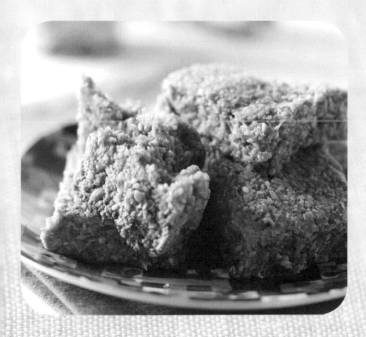

71

SOYBEANS

A valuable bean, rich in minerals and disease-preventing plant chemicals, soybeans are a complete source of protein and an ideal food for vegetarians.

Soybeans have been cultivated in China for over 10,000 years and are among the few plant sources of complete protein, containing all eight essential amino acids needed in our diet. Soy is also an excellent source of calcium, B vitamins, potassium, zinc, and magnesium. It is a very rich source of iron, although this iron may only be absorbed by the body if consumed with vitamin C-rich foods. Soy is rich in plant chemicals that offer protection from diseases, including breast and prostate cancers and heart disease. A regular intake of soybeans can also reduce menopausal symptoms.

- Complete source of low saturated fat protein.
- Rich in plant compounds, which may help protect against hormone-based cancers.
- Help lower "bad" cholesterol and protect against heart disease.
- Can reduce symptoms of the menopause, including hot flushes.

Practical tips:
Canned soybeans are a quick and easy alternative to dried beans and contain a similar nutritional profile. Use beans in soups and casseroles, mash for a dip, or add to vegetable burgers. Tofu is made from processed soybeans and is a good low-fat, low-sodium alternative. Some of the wheat flour in baking recipes can be replaced with soy flour to increase nutrient content.

DID YOU KNOW?

Edamame is the name for fresh soybeans, which you can find ready podded, frozen, or, sometimes, fresh in delis and markets. Cook and use them as you would fava beans and other fresh legumes.

MAJOR NUTRIENTS PER 2¼ oz/60 G DRIED SOYBEANS

Kcalories	250
Total fat	12 g
Protein	22 g
Carbohydrate	18 g
Fiber	5.6 g
Folate	225 mcg
Vitamin B1	0.5 mg
Riboflavin	0.5 mg
Niacin	0.95 mg
Magnesium	168 mg
Potassium	1078 mg
Zinc	2.9 g
Calcium	166 mg
Iron	9.4 mg

Marinated soybeans

SERVES 10–12

*8 oz/225 g fresh soybeans,
washed, and stalks trimmed
with scissors*
1¼ cups Chinese rice wine
generous ¾ cup cold water
3 tbsp sugar

Method

1 Cook the beans in a covered saucepan of lightly salted, boiling water for about 15 minutes, or until they begin to soften but not open up. Drain and cool.
2 Place the beans in a large bowl and pour over the rest of the ingredients, immersing the beans. Leave for 24 hours in a cool place. Serve cold, and pod the beans before eating.

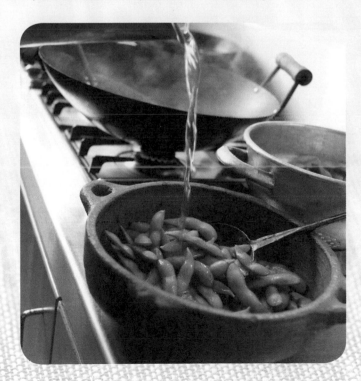

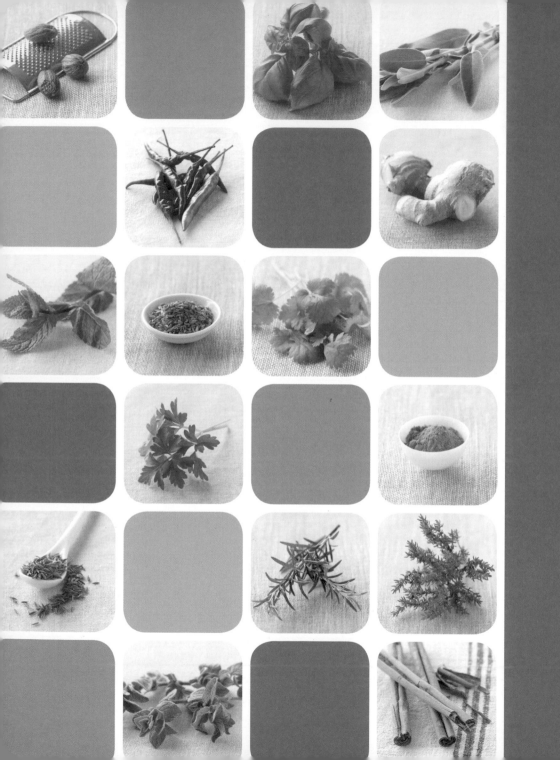

HERBS AND SPICES

Offering both nutritional and medicinal benefits, herbs and spices, even in small quantities, can make a big impact on any diet. Use them to top a favorite pasta dish or curry, or bake them into delicious breads or muffins.

(**V**) Suitable for vegetarians

(**D**) Ideal for dieters

(**P**) Suitable for pregnancy

(**C**) Suitable for children over 5 years

(**Q**) Quick to prepare and cook

72

BASIL

The highly fragrant, bright green leaves of basil are mildly sedative and pain relieving, and can help beat indigestion.

Basil is perhaps best known as the major ingredient in the Italian sauce pesto. Yet the herb has been used for thousands of years in India and the Mediterranean, has several health benefits, and has long been used in traditional herbal medicine as a remedy for indigestion, nausea, and stomach ache. It is mildly sedative and an infusion of basil oil can even be used as an insect repellent and to offer sting relief. Basil contains strongly antioxidant flavonoid compounds. The leaves contain volatile oils that contain chemicals to fight food poisoning bacteria. The chemical eugenol, also present, is an anti-inflammatory similar to aspirin and can help relieve the pain of arthritis and may ease irritable bowel syndrome.

- Traditionally used in remedies for indigestion, nausea, and stomach ache.
- Acts as an insect repellent and has antibacterial action.
- Anti-inflammatory.
- High in lutein and zeaxanthin for eye health.

Practical tips:
Basil is best added at the end of cooking to preserve its flavor, aroma, and oils. Basil leaves, if large, should be torn rather than cut with a knife. To make a quick pesto, crush basil with pine nuts, olive oil, salt, and pepper and use to dress pasta. Sprinkle basil over a salad of tomatoes and mozzarella.

DID YOU KNOW?
The chemical estragole, found in basil, has been linked with cancer in animals, but there is no risk to humans even if huge amounts are eaten.

MAJOR NUTRIENTS PER ½ oz/15 g BASIL

Kcalories	222
Total fat	1.8 g
Protein	5 g
Carbohydrate	46 g
Fiber	3.6 g
Niacin	3 mg
Vitamin B1	0.2 mg
Vitamin B6	0.3 mg
Selenium	19.6 mcg
Magnesium	86 mg
Iron	0.8 mg
Zinc	1.3 g
Calcium	20 mg
Lutein/Zeaxanthin	848 mcg

Pepper and basil pots

SERVES 4

1 tsp olive oil
2 shallots, finely chopped
2 garlic cloves, crushed
2 red bell peppers, peeled, seeded,
*   and sliced into strips*
1 orange bell pepper, peeled,
*   seeded, and sliced into strips*
4 tomatoes, thinly sliced
2 tbsp shredded fresh basil
pepper
salad greens, to serve

Method

1 Lightly brush 4 ramekin dishes with the oil. Mix the shallots and garlic together in a bowl and season with pepper to taste.

2 Layer the red and orange bell peppers with the tomatoes in the prepared ramekin dishes, sprinkling each layer with the shallot mixture and shredded basil. When all the ingredients have been added, cover lightly with plastic wrap or parchment paper. Weigh down using small weights and leave in the refrigerator for at least 6 hours, or preferably overnight.

3 When ready to serve, remove the weights and carefully run a knife around the edges. Invert onto serving plates and serve with salad greens.

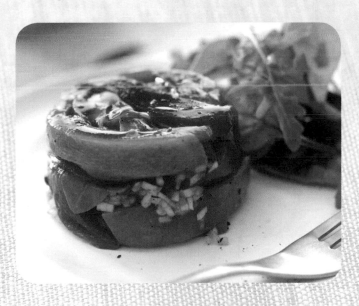

73 MINT

Popular as a garden herb, mint is a remedy to calm and relax the stomach, and can relieve travel sickness and the congestion of colds.

For thousands of years, mint has been used for its flavor as well as its medicinal purposes. The three main types of mint commonly used are peppermint, spearmint, and apple mint. The menthol oils that they contain, particularly peppermint, are a natural remedy for indigestion, which is why mint tea is traditionally consumed after a rich meal. Menthol can also clear head and chest congestion during colds and flu, and for people who suffer from allergic rhinitis. The oils are antibacterial and may help prevent *H.pylori*, which causes stomach ulcers, and food poisoning bugs salmonella and *E.coli*, from multiplying. Mint contains plant chemicals, which have been shown to block the growth of certain cancers in animals.

- Relieves indigestion and calms the stomach.
- Relieves nasal and chest congestion.
- Contains antibacterial properties.
- May have anticancer action.

Practical tips:
Mint is best enjoyed fresh as the dried leaves lose much of their potency. A simple way to enjoy fresh mint is to chop it finely and mix with plain yogurt to serve with lamb or eggplant. Make an easy mint sauce by combining fresh chopped mint with balsamic vinegar. You can also steep a handful of fresh leaves in boiling water for 5 minutes to make a mint tea—strain before drinking.

DID YOU KNOW?

If you put a few stalks of freshly picked mint in a jar of water, within a few days they will grow roots, which can be planted indoors for a year-round supply.

MAJOR NUTRIENTS PER ½ oz/15 g MINT

Kcalories	7
Total fat	Trace
Protein	0.5 g
Carbohydrate	1.2 g
Fiber	1 g
Folate	16 mcg
Magnesium	9 mg
Potassium	69 mg
Calcium	30 mg
Iron	1.8 mg

Mint and spinach chutney

SERVES 4–6

2 oz/55 g tender fresh
   spinach leaves

3 tbsp fresh mint leaves

2 tbsp chopped fresh cilantro
   leaves

1 small red onion,
   coarsely chopped

1 small garlic clove, chopped

1 fresh green chile, chopped
   (seeded, if liked)

2½ tsp sugar

1 tbsp tamarind juice or juice
   of ½ lemon

Method

1 Place all the ingredients in a food processor and process until smooth, adding only as much water as necessary to enable the blades to move.

2 Transfer to a serving bowl, cover, and let chill in the refrigerator for at least 30 minutes before serving. Serve with samosas or lamb kebobs.

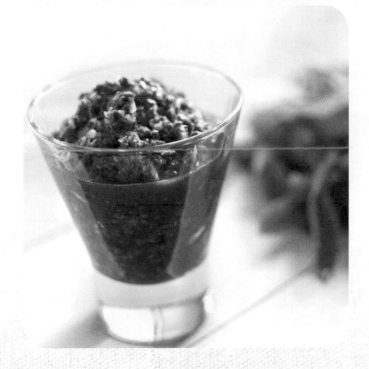

74

PARSLEY

A traditional herbal remedy, parsley is strongly antioxidant and anticoagulant, and is also rich in vitamin C and iron.

Flat-leaf and curly-leaf parsley both have a similar nutritional profile. Parsley sprigs are often simply used as a garnish and then discarded, which is a pity as the leaves are a good source of several nutrients including vitamin C and iron. Myristicin, a compound found in parsley, inhibits tumors in animals and has a strong antioxidant action, neutralizing carcinogens in the body, such as the dangerous compounds in tobacco smoke and barbecue smoke. Parsley is also an anticoagulant, and contains compounds of oils that are linked with relief from menstrual problems such as pain, fluid retention, and cramps.

- A good source of vitamin C and iron, potassium, and folate.
- Source of lutein and zeaxanthin to prevent macular degeneration.
- A breath purifier.
- Antioxidant and anticancer action.
- Contains the essential oil apiol used as a traditional remedy for fluid retention and menstrual disorders.

Practical tips:
Picked parsley keeps well for several days in the refrigerator in a plastic bag. Combine plenty of chopped parsley with mint, lemon juice, and oil and toss with cooked bulgur wheat to make tabbouleh. Make a flat-leaf parsley pesto with ground walnuts and olive oil for pasta.

DID YOU KNOW?

Parsley is a member of Umbelliferae family of plants and is closely related to parsnip. There is a "root parsley" that can be used in a similar way and is popular in European cooking.

MAJOR NUTRIENTS PER ½ OZ/15 G PARSLEY

Kcalories	5
Total fat	Trace
Protein	0.5 g
Carbohydrate	1 g
Fiber	0.5 g
Vitamin C	20 mg
Folate	23 mcg
Magnesium	8 mg
Potassium	83 mg
Calcium	21 mg
Iron	0.9 mg
Beta-carotene	758 mcg
Lutein/Zeaxanthin	834 mcg

Parsley vinaigrette

MAKES ABOUT ⅔ CUP (v) (D) (P) (c) (Q)

½ cup olive oil

3 tbsp white wine vinegar or
　lemon juice

1½ tbsp chopped fresh parsley

1 tsp Dijon mustard

½ tsp superfine sugar

salt and pepper

Method

1 Place all the ingredients in a screw-top jar, secure the lid, and shake vigorously until a thick emulsion forms. Taste and adjust the seasoning, if necessary.

2 Use at once or store in an airtight container in the refrigerator for up to 3 days. Serve as a dressing for any green salad. Always whisk or shake the dressing before using, and strain through a nonmetallic strainer if the herbs begin to darken.

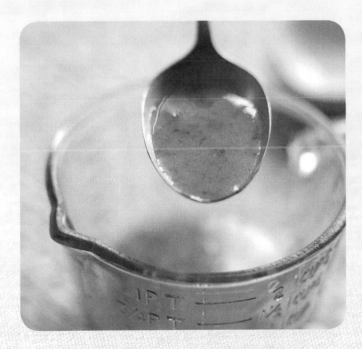

75 ROSEMARY

Pungent fresh rosemary has strong medicinal benefits, can fight the symptoms of colds and flu, and help prevent diseases of aging.

Traditionally, rosemary has been used as a mental stimulant, memory booster, general tonic, and to aid circulation. An infusion of rosemary tea has long been recommended by herbalists to treat colds, flu, and rheumatism. Like several other herbs, rosemary has been shown to fight bacteria that can cause throat infections such as *E.coli*, and *staphylococcus*, so an infusion of rosemary makes a good gargle. In addition, recent research has found that rosemary is one of the leading herbs for its antioxidant activity, helping to reduce the risk of diseases and aging effects.

- Strong antioxidant activity.
- Memory and brain booster.
- Contains antibacterial properties.
- Used as a general tonic and may lift depression.

Practical tips:
Rosemary dries well and retains some of its antioxidant effects. Hang sprigs up to dry in a warm kitchen then remove the leaves and store in an airtight container. Fresh rosemary leaves can be chopped and mixed with thyme, sage, and oregano and added to Mediterranean casseroles or omelet fillings. Use fresh sprigs with garlic to season roast chicken, lamb, and pork. When making bread, add some chopped fresh leaves to the mix.

DID YOU KNOW?

In tests, rosemary extract (rather than fresh or dried leaves) has been found to act as a detoxifier for the liver, to help boost skin condition, and to block estrogens in the body in a similar way to anti-breast cancer drugs.

MAJOR NUTRIENTS PER ½ OZ/15 G ROSEMARY

Kcalories	20
Total fat	0.9 g
Protein	0.5 g
Carbohydrate	3.1 g
Fiber	2 g
Folate	16 mcg
Magnesium	14 mg
Potassium	100 mg
Calcium	48 mg
Iron	1 mg

Monkfish, rosemary, and turkey bacon skewers

MAKES 12

9 oz/250 g monkfish fillet
12 fresh rosemary stalks, plus fresh
   sprigs, to garnish
3 tbsp Spanish olive oil
juice of ½ small lemon
1 garlic clove, crushed
6 thick slices turkey bacon
salt and pepper
lemon wedges, to serve

Aïoli

3 egg yolks
4 fresh garlic cloves
juice of ½ lemon
⅔ cup extra virgin olive oil
1 level tsp mustard powder

Method

1 Slice the monkfish fillets in half
lengthwise, then cut each fillet
into 12 bite-size chunks to
make a total of 24 pieces.
Place the monkfish pieces in
a large bowl.

2 To prepare the rosemary
skewers, strip the leaves off
the stalks and set them aside,
leaving a few leaves at one
end. Finely chop the reserved
leaves and whisk together in a
bowl with the oil, lemon juice,
garlic, salt, and pepper. Add
the monkfish pieces and toss
until coated in the marinade.

Cover and let marinate in the
refrigerator for 1–2 hours.

3 Preheat the broiler or
barbecue. To make the aïoli,
place all the ingredients except
the oil in a food processor and
process until mixed. With the
motor still running, pour the oil
through the feed tube until it
forms a thick sauce. Transfer
to a bowl and set aside.

4 Cut each turkey bacon slice in
half lengthwise, then in half
widthwise, and roll up each
piece. Thread 2 pieces of
monkfish alternately with
2 bacon rolls onto each
rosemary skewer.

5 Cook under the preheated
broiler or over hot coals for
10 minutes, or until cooked,
turning occasionally and
basting with any remaining
marinade. Be careful that the
skewers do not burn. Serve
with lemon wedges and aïoli.

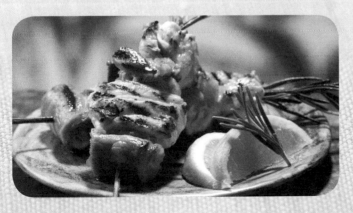

76 SAGE

Rich in beneficial compounds, sage helps to slow down the aging process and minimize symptoms of arthritis and asthma.

Native to the Mediterranean, sage has been used for thousands of years and has one of the longest histories of use of any medicinal herb. It contains a variety of volatile oils, flavonoids, and phenolic acids. Sage is in the top ten of herbs that have the most powerful antioxidant effect, neutralizing the cell-damaging free radicals that are thought to be linked with the aging process. Herbalists have long believed that sage is an outstanding memory enhancer and in trials, even small amounts significantly improved short-term recall. Sage is also antibacterial and can help reduce the number of hot flushes in menopausal women, and is recommended for people with inflammatory conditions such as rheumatoid arthritis and asthma.

- Strongly antioxidant, antibacterial, and preservative.
- Boosts memory.
- Reduces hot flushes in many menopausal women.
- Has anti-inflammatory properties.

Practical tips:
Sage is an easy-to-grow, perennial hardy shrub available throughout the year. The leaves can be dried by laying them on a rack in a warm, dry place and then stored in an airtight tin. Add sage to other chopped herbs for a herb omelet or stuffing. Sprinkle chopped fresh sage on pizzas and pasta.

DID YOU KNOW?

For a long time herbalists have recognized sage's antioxidant qualities. The Ancient Greeks used it to help preserve meat, while tenth-century physicians in Arabia believed it helped promote immortality.

MAJOR NUTRIENTS PER ½ oz/15 g SAGE

Kcalories	22
Total fat	0.9 g
Protein	0.7 g
Carbohydrate	4.2 g
Fiber	2.8 g
Folate	19 mcg
Magnesium	30 mg
Potassium	75 mg
Calcium	116 mg
Iron	1.9 mg
Beta-carotene	244 mcg

Garlic and sage bread

MAKES I LOAF

1¾ cups strong whole wheat
    bread flour, plus extra
    for dusting
1 package active dry yeast
3 tbsp chopped fresh sage, plus
    fresh leaves, to garnish
1 tsp sea salt
3 garlic cloves, finely chopped
1 tsp honey
⅔ cup lukewarm water
canola oil, for brushing
low-fat cream cheese, to serve

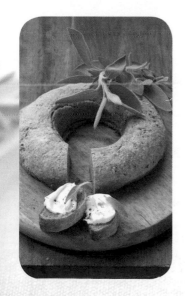

Method

1 Sift the flour into a bowl and tip in the bran from the strainer. Stir in the yeast, sage, and salt. Set aside 1 teaspoon of the garlic and stir the remainder into the bowl. Make a well in the center and pour in the honey and water. Stir well until the dough begins to come together, then knead with your hands until it leaves the side of the bowl. Turn out onto a lightly floured surface and knead for 10 minutes, or until smooth and elastic.

2 Brush a bowl with oil. Shape the dough into a ball, place it in the bowl, and place the bowl into a plastic bag or cover with a damp dish towel. Let rise in a warm place for 1 hour, or until the dough has doubled in volume.

3 Brush a baking sheet with oil. Turn out the dough onto a lightly floured surface, knock back with your fist, and knead for 2 minutes. Roll the dough into a long sausage, shape into a ring, and place it onto the baking sheet. Brush the outside of a bowl with oil and place it in the center of the ring to prevent it from closing up while the dough is rising. Place the baking sheet into a plastic bag or cover with a damp dish towel and leave in a warm place for 30 minutes.

4 Preheat the oven to 400°F/200°C. Remove the bowl from the center of the loaf. Sprinkle the loaf with the reserved garlic and a little flour and bake in the preheated oven for 25–30 minutes, until golden brown and the loaf sounds hollow when tapped on the base with your knuckles. Transfer to a wire rack to cool. Cut into slices, spread with cream cheese, garnish with sage leaves, and serve.

77

OREGANO

Pungent oregano is the herb highest in antioxidant activity, helping to prevent food poisoning bacteria and boost the immune system.

According to tests carried out by the United States Department of Agriculture, oregano has more antioxidant activity than any other herb. The herb has demonstrated forty-two times more antioxidant activity than apples, twelve times more than oranges, and four times more than blueberries. The volatile oils in this spice include thymol and carvacrol, which have both been shown to strongly inhibit the growth of bacteria, including *staphylococcus aureus*. Oregano is also a good source of several nutrients, including calcium, potassium, iron, and magnesium. It is also high in dietary fiber and may help lower "bad" cholesterol.

- One of the most powerful antioxidant plants.
- Antibacterial and may relieve the symptoms of colds.
- Rich in minerals.
- High in fiber and may aid digestion.

DID YOU KNOW?

When replacing fresh oregano with dried leaves in a recipe, reduce the amount you use by about half.

MAJOR NUTRIENTS PER ½ oz/15 G OREGANO

Kcalories	21
Total fat	0.8 g
Protein	0.7 g
Carbohydrate	4.5 g
Fiber	3 g
Niacin	0.4 mg
Folate	19 mcg
Magnesium	19 mg
Potassium	117 mg
Calcium	110 mg
Iron	3 mg
Beta-carotene	288 mcg

Practical tips:
Oregano is an easy-to-grow herb and can be kept in a pot on the windowsill. The leaves dry well and can be stored in an airtight container. Replace dried oregano at least every 3 months as it loses its aroma and flavor over time. Oregano is one of the traditional herbs to include in mixed herbs and herbes de Provence. Oregano marries particularly well with eggs, tomatoes, lamb, and chicken.

Tuna with green sauce

SERVES 4 (**D**) (**C**) (**Q**)

4 fresh tuna steaks, about ¾ inch/
   2 cm thick

olive oil, for brushing

salt and pepper

lemon wedges, to serve

Green sauce

2 oz/55 g fresh flat-leaf parsley,
   leaves and stems

4 scallions, chopped

2 garlic cloves, chopped

3 anchovy fillets in oil, drained

1 oz/30 g fresh basil leaves

½ tbsp capers in brine, rinsed
   and dried

2 fresh oregano sprigs or ½ tsp
   dried oregano

½ cup extra virgin olive oil, plus
   extra if necessary

1–2 tbsp lemon juice, or to taste

Method

1 To make the green sauce, place the parsley, scallions, garlic,
   anchovy fillets, basil, capers, and oregano in a food processor and
   pulse to chop and blend together. With the motor still running, pour
   the oil through the feed tube. Add lemon juice to taste, then process
   again. If the sauce is too thick, add a little extra oil. Transfer to a
   bowl, cover, and let chill in the refrigerator until needed.

2 Place a cast-iron griddle pan over high heat until you can feel the
   heat rising from the surface. Brush the tuna steaks with oil and
   place, oiled-side down, on the hot pan and cook for 2 minutes.

3 Lightly brush the top side of the tuna steaks with a little more oil.
   Use a pair of tongs to turn over the tuna steaks, then season with
   salt and pepper to taste. Continue cooking for an additional
   2 minutes for rare or for up to 4 minutes for well done.

4 Transfer the tuna steaks to serving plates and serve with the green
   sauce spooned over, accompanied by lemon wedges.

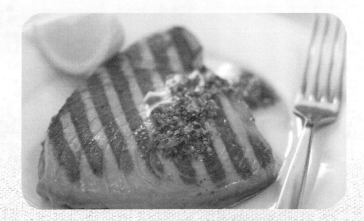

78

CILANTRO

The leaves of cilantro are antibacterial, anti-inflammatory, and can significantly improve the blood cholesterol profile.

Cilantro has a reputation for being high on the list of the healing herbs. Research has shown that when cilantro was added to the diet of diabetic mice, it helped stimulate their secretion of insulin and lowered their blood sugar. The leaves contain the compound dodecenal, which tests show is twice as effective at killing salmonella bacteria as some antibiotics. In addition, eight other antibiotic compounds were isolated from the plant. Cilantro has also been shown to lower "bad" cholesterol and increase "good" cholesterol. It is a good source of several nutrients, including potassium and calcium, and contains high levels of lutein and zeaxanthin, which help protect our eyes and eyesight.

- Regulates blood sugars and therefore may help diabetics and people who are insulin-resistant.
- Anti-inflammatory and antibacterial.
- Has a positive impact on blood cholesterol levels.
- May contribute to improved eye health.

Practical tips:
Use fresh cilantro as it loses most of its aroma and flavor when dried. The leaves are very delicate so store carefully, well wrapped, or use leaves from a growing plant. Fresh cilantro should be added to cooked dishes, such as curries, at the last minute, as once cooked it loses aroma and flavor.

DID YOU KNOW?

Leaves of fresh cilantro bear a strong resemblance to Italian flat-leaf parsley—they both belong to the same plant family, *umbelliferae*.

MAJOR NUTRIENTS PER ½ oz/15 g CILANTRO

Kcalories	3
Total fat	Trace
Protein	0.3 g
Carbohydrate	0.5 g
Fiber	0.4 g
Folate	9 mcg
Potassium	78 mg
Calcium	10 mg
Iron	0.3 mg
Beta-carotene	590 mcg
Lutein/Zeaxanthin	130 mcg

Green leaf and herb jam with olives

SERVES 4 (V) (D) (P) (C)

8 oz/225 g fresh baby
   spinach leaves

handful of celery leaves

3 tbsp olive oil

2–3 garlic cloves, crushed

1 tsp cumin seeds

6–8 black olives, pitted and finely
   chopped

1 large bunch of fresh flat-leaf
   parsley leaves, finely chopped

1 large bunch of fresh cilantro
   leaves, finely chopped

1 tsp Spanish smoked paprika

juice of ½ lemon

salt and pepper

toasted flat bread or crusty bread
   and black olives, to serve

Method

1 Place the spinach and celery leaves in a steamer and steam until tender. Refresh the leaves under cold running water, drain well, and squeeze out the excess water. Place the steamed leaves on a wooden cutting board and chop to a pulp.

2 Heat 2 tablespoons of the oil in a tagine or heavy-bottom casserole. Add the garlic and cumin seeds, then cook over medium heat for 1–2 minutes, stirring, until they emit a nutty aroma. Stir in the olives with the parsley and cilantro and add the paprika.

3 Toss in the pulped spinach and celery and cook over low heat, stirring occasionally, for 10 minutes, until the mixture is smooth and compact. Season with salt and pepper to taste and let cool.

4 Tip the mixture into a bowl and bind with the remaining oil and the lemon juice. Serve with toasted flat bread or crusty bread and olives.

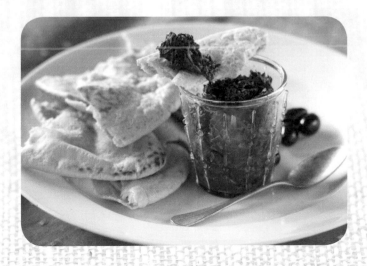

79

THYME

This herb may be tiny but, with an antioxidant action in the top ten of all herbs, it packs a huge health punch.

The evergreen leaves of thyme have a powerful, aromatic flavor and strong antioxidant action because of the volatile oils and plant compounds they contain. The most important of these is thymol oil. Research on this oil has found it can boost the effects of healthy omega-3 fats on the body, for example, the omega-3 DHA found in fish oils, which has been shown to be important for healthy brain function. The oils in thyme are strongly antibacterial and can protect us against food poisoning bugs such as *E.coli*, *bacillus*, and *staphylococcus*. Lastly they are rich in flavonoids, which protect us against the diseases of aging, and they are a good source of vitamin C and iron.

- Boosts omega-3 fats' actions in the body.
- May boost brain power.
- Strongly antiseptic and antibiotic.
- Rich in flavonoid antioxidants, vitamin C, and iron.

Practical tips:
Fresh stalks can be tied with bay leaves and parsley to make a simple bouquet garni for fish soups and stews. Add chopped fresh thyme leaves, mint, and parsley to an omelet for wonderful flavor and aroma. Stuff a roasting chicken with plenty of thyme or lemon thyme. If necessary, the easiest way to remove leaves from stalks is with a fork.

DID YOU KNOW?
Thyme oil has been used since the Middle Ages for its antiseptic properties, and is often recommended by herbalists today as a treatment for bronchitis or a mouthwash.

MAJOR NUTRIENTS PER ½ oz/15 g THYME

Kcalories	15
Total fat	0.2 g
Protein	0.8 g
Carbohydrate	3.6 g
Fiber	2.1 g
Vitamin C	24 mg
Calcium	61 mg
Potassium	91 mg
Iron	2.6 mg
Zinc	0.3 mg
Beta-carotene	428 mcg

Thyme, rosemary, and lemon oil

MAKES GENEROUS 1 CUP

*10–15 fresh thyme sprigs (each
    about 5 inches/13 cm long)*
*5 fresh rosemary sprigs (each
    about 5 inches/13 cm long)*
zest of 2 lemons
generous 1 cup canola oil

Method

1 Preheat the oven to 300°F/150°C. Remove the leaves from the
   thyme and rosemary sprigs. Cut the lemon zest into strips.

2 Pour the oil into an ovenproof glass dish and add the leaves and
   lemon zest strips. Place the dish in the center of the preheated oven
   and heat for 1½–2 hours.

3 If you have a digital thermometer, test the oil. It should reach a
   temperature of 250°F/120°C before you remove it from the oven.
   Let cool for at least 30 minutes. Store the oil in the refrigerator as
   it is, or strain through cheesecloth and let chill in the refrigerator
   until needed. Serve with slices of crusty bread.

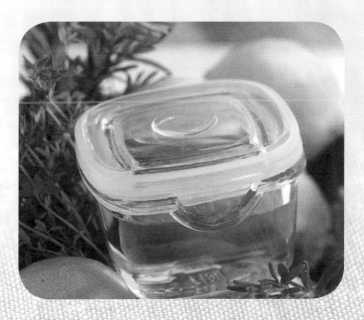

80 FENNEL SEEDS

Anise-flavored fennel seeds have an appetite-suppressant effect, making them useful for dieters. They may also calm the digestive system.

Fennel seeds come from both the fennel herb and the fennel vegetable bulb. They have long been regarded as an aid to weight loss because they are said to reduce appetite when consumed as fennel tea. Chewing them is a remedy for bad breath. For women, fennel seeds are helpful when breastfeeding, as they contain compounds that mimic estrogen and therefore stimulate milk production. As an infusion, it can treat flatulence, colic in babies, and stomach cramps. However, the seeds should be avoided during pregnancy as they may overstimulate the uterus. Fennel seeds may also be good for relieving menopausal symptoms.

• May help control appetite.
• Remedy for halitosis.
• Digestive aid and cure for flatulence and colic.
• Stimulate milk production when breastfeeding.

Practical tips:
Make a fennel tea by steeping a spoonful of seeds in boiling water for 5 minutes, then strain. Fennel seeds are delicious with pork so make slits in the meat and stuff with a few seeds before roasting. Fennel flavors also go particularly well with fish and can be added by putting crushed seeds, olive oil, and chopped tomatoes over the top of white fish before baking. Add extra flavor to potato salad with crushed fennel seeds.

DID YOU KNOW?

Highly respected as both a food and a medicine in ancient Rome and Greece, fennel was also thought to have magical powers in medieval times—the seeds were inserted in keyholes to protect the home from ghosts.

MAJOR NUTRIENTS PER 1 oz /15 g FENNEL SEEDS

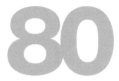

Kcalories	20
Total fat	0.9 g
Protein	0.9 g
Carbohydrate	3 g
Fiber	2.3 g
Calcium	69 mg
Potassium	98 mg
Magnesium	22 mg
Iron	1 mg

Fish skewers

MAKES 8

pinch of saffron threads, pounded
1 tbsp hot skim milk
⅓ cup low-fat plain yogurt
1 tbsp garlic puree
1 tbsp ginger puree
½ tsp salt (optional)
½ tsp sugar
juice of ½ lemon
½–1 tsp chili powder
½ tsp garam masala
1 tsp ground fennel seeds
2 tsp chickpea flour
1 lb 10 oz/750 g salmon fillets,
*   skinned and cut into 2-inch/*
*   5-cm cubes*
3 tbsp olive oil, plus extra
*   for brushing*
sliced tomatoes and sliced
*   cucumber, to garnish*
lemon wedges, to serve

Method

1 Soak the pounded saffron in the hot milk for 10 minutes.

2 Place all the remaining ingredients, except the fish and oil, in a bowl and beat with a fork or a wire whisk until smooth. Stir in the saffron and milk, mix well, and add the fish cubes. Using a metal spoon, mix gently, turning the fish around until fully coated with the marinade. Cover and let marinate in the refrigerator for 2 hours. Return to room temperature before cooking.

3 Preheat the broiler to high. Brush the broiler rack generously with oil and 8 metal skewers lightly with oil. Line the broiler pan with foil. Thread the fish onto the prepared skewers, leaving a narrow gap between each piece. Arrange on the broiler rack and cook 4 inches/10 cm below the heat source for 3 minutes. Brush half the 3 tablespoons of oil over the kebabs and cook

for an additional 1 minute. Turn over and brush any remaining marinade over the fish. Cook for 3 minutes. Brush the remaining oil over the fish and cook for an additional 2 minutes, or until the fish is lightly charred.

4 Remove from the heat and let rest for 5 minutes. Garnish with tomato and cucumber slices and serve with lemon wedges.

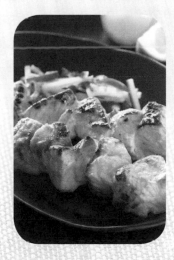

81

CHILES

Fiery chiles pack a nutritional and flavorful punch and research shows that they are one of the healthiest spices available.

The heat that chiles add to a dish comes from a compound called capsaicin, which is known to relieve the pain and inflammation associated with arthritis. Capsaicin also appears to block production of cancerous cells in prostate cancer, and to act as an anticoagulant to help protect against blood clots that can cause heart attacks or strokes. Red chiles also contain high levels of carotenes. Chile consumption also helps lower the amount of insulin required to lower blood sugar after a meal and thus could be of help to diabetics and people with insulin resistance. Chiles may also increase the metabolic rate slightly, which could help with weight loss.

- Contain capsaicin, which can relieve pain and inflammation associated with arthritis.
- Strongly antioxidant to help beat the effects of aging diseases.
- Help lower "bad" cholesterol and reduce risk of blood clots.
- Rich in vitamin C and carotenes to boost the immune system.

Practical tips:
There are hundreds of types of chiles in various shapes, colors, and degrees of heat. Don't rub eyes when preparing chiles—you can wear thin disposable gloves when handling. Dried peppers and chili powders should be kept in a dark, airtight jar.

DID YOU KNOW?

Chiles are said to improve psoriasis and shingles when topically applied in a cream.

MAJOR NUTRIENTS PER 1 oz/30 g CHILE

Kcalories	12
Total fat	trace
Protein	0.5 g
Carbohydrate	2.6 g
Fiber	0.4 g
Folate	0.4 g
Vitamin C	43 mg
Niacin	0.4 mg
Potassium	97 mg
Iron	0.3 mg
Beta-carotene	160 mcg
Lutein/Zeaxanthin	213 mcg

Shrimp with coconut milk, chile, and curry leaf

SERVES 4　(**D**)(**P**)(**C**)(**Q**)

4 tbsp olive oil

½ tsp black or brown mustard seeds

½ tsp fenugreek seeds

1 large onion, finely chopped

2 tsp garlic puree

2 tsp ginger puree

1–2 fresh green chiles, chopped and seeded

1 tbsp ground coriander

½ tsp ground turmeric

½ tsp chili powder

1 tsp salt, or to taste

generous 1 cup canned low-fat coconut milk

1 lb/450 g cooked peeled jumbo shrimp, thawed and drained if frozen

1 tbsp tamarind juice or juice of ½ lime

½ tsp crushed black pepper

10–12 fresh or dried curry leaves

Method

1 Heat 3 tablespoons of the oil in a medium saucepan over medium–high heat. When hot but not smoking, add the mustard seeds, followed by the fenugreek seeds and the onion. Cook, stirring frequently, for 5–6 minutes, until the onion is soft but not brown. Add the garlic and ginger purees, and the chiles and cook, stirring frequently, for an additional 5–6 minutes, until the onion is a light golden color.

2 Add the coriander, turmeric, and chili powder and cook, stirring for 1 minute. Add the salt and coconut milk, followed by the shrimp and tamarind juice. Bring to a slow simmer and cook, stirring occasionally, for 3–4 minutes.

3 Meanwhile, heat the remaining 1 tablespoon of oil in a very small saucepan over medium heat. Add the pepper and curry leaves and cook for 20–25 seconds, then fold the aromatic oil into the shrimp mixture. Remove from the heat and serve immediately.

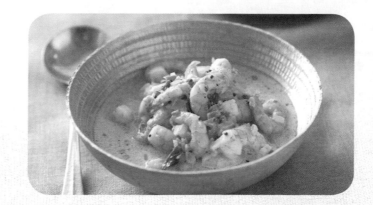

82

CINNAMON

Sweet cinnamon is an anti-inflammatory, antibacterial spice that can help relieve bloating and heartburn, and offer protection against strokes.

Cinnamon contains several volatile oils and compounds, including cinnamaldehyde, cinnamyl acetate, and cinnamyl alcohol, which have a variety of beneficial actions. Cinnamaldehyde has an anticoagulant action, meaning that it can help to protect against strokes, and is also anti-inflammatory, relieving symptoms of arthritis and asthma. The spice is a digestive aid, relieving bloating and flatulence, and it can reduce the discomfort of heartburn. Cinnamon has antibacterial action that can block the yeast fungus, candida, and bugs that can cause food poisoning. In one study, cinnamon was shown to lower blood sugars and blood cholesterol.

- Helps to beat indigestion and bloating.
- Antibacterial and antifungal.
- Helps prevent blood clots.
- May lower "bad" cholesterol and blood sugars.

Practical tips:
Whole bark cinnamon sticks will retain their flavor and aroma for a year, while the ground dried spice will last for about six months. You can tell if ground cinnamon is still fresh by sniffing it—if it has lost its aroma then you need to discard it. Whole or part sticks can be added to apple or pear fruit compotes and to mulled wine. Ground cinnamon is a good addition to a curry.

DID YOU KNOW?

True cinnamon is the inner bark of an evergreen tree of the laurel family native to Sri Lanka, and cassia is another variety native to China. Both are widely available, but it is not always possible to know which one you are buying.

MAJOR NUTRIENTS PER ½ oz/15 g CINNAMON

Kcalories	18
Total fat	Trace
Protein	Trace
Carbohydrate	5.5 g
Fiber	3.7 g
Folate	287 mcg
Potassium	34 mg
Calcium	84 mg
Iron	2.6 mg

Broiled cinnamon oranges

SERVES 8

4 large oranges
1 tsp ground cinnamon
1 tbsp raw brown sugar

Method

1 Preheat the broiler to high. Cut the oranges in half and discard any seeds. Using a sharp or curved grapefruit knife, carefully cut the flesh away from the skin by cutting around the edge of the fruit. Cut across the segments to loosen the flesh into bite-size pieces that will then spoon out easily.

2 Arrange the orange halves, cut-side up, in a shallow, ovenproof dish. Mix the cinnamon and sugar together in a small bowl and sprinkle evenly over the orange halves.

3 Cook under the preheated broiler for 3–5 minutes, or until the sugar has caramelized and is golden and bubbling. Serve immediately.

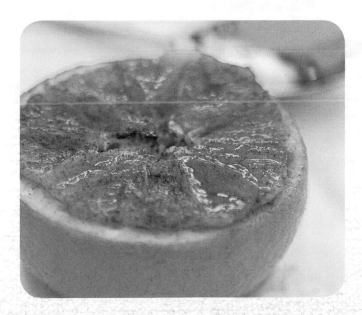

83 CUMIN SEEDS

With its antiseptic action, cumin offers sore throat relief, and helps the digestive system to work efficiently.

Small, brown cumin seeds are harvested from a herb belonging to the parsley family. Its flavor is warm and spicy but not too hot. The spice has been used since ancient times—the Romans used it as an appetizer and digestive. Research has shown this to be true as cumin stimulates the secretion of pancreatic enzymes necessary for efficient digestion and nutrient absorption. Currently, cumin is being investigated for its antioxidant powers and it may help to block cancer growth. The seeds are rich in iron. Cumin is an antiseptic so an infusion of cumin seeds with honey makes an ideal drink for people with a sore throat.

- Aid digestion.
- May help prevent cancers.
- Contain antiseptic properties.
- Rich in iron for healthy blood.

Practical tips:
Buy whole seeds as these retain their aroma longer than ground cumin. All dried spices are best kept in airtight containers in cool, dry, dark conditions. Use opaque containers to store spices on racks as they deteriorate rapidly in light. Add lightly ground cumin seeds to brown rice and chopped dried fruits and nuts for a delicious salad. Cumin also goes well with beans, such as lentils and chickpeas.

DID YOU KNOW?

Cumin seeds are native to the Middle East but have been cultivated in India and China for thousands of years, and are one of the key ingredients of curry blends.

MAJOR NUTRIENTS PER ½ oz/15 G CUMIN SEEDS

Kcalories	23
Total fat	1 g
Protein	1 g
Carbohydrate	2.6 g
Fiber	0.6 g
Calcium	56 mg
Magnesium	22 mg
Potassium	107 mg
Iron	4 mg

Carrot and cumin soup

SERVES 1–2

1 medium–large carrot, peeled
   and finely chopped
1 small garlic clove, chopped
1 medium–large shallot,
   finely chopped
1 ripe tomato, peeled
   and chopped
½ tsp ground cumin
generous ¾ cup vegetable stock
1 bouquet garni
2 tsp dry sherry
pepper
1 tbsp low-fat Greek-style yogurt
   and a pinch of cumin, to serve

Method

1 Place all the ingredients except the sherry and yogurt in a saucepan with a lid. Bring to simmering point over high heat, then reduce the heat and simmer for 30 minutes, or until the vegetables are tender. Remove the pan from the heat and let cool slightly. Remove the bouquet garni.

2 Pour the soup into a food processor or blender and process until smooth. Return to the saucepan, add the sherry, and reheat. Taste and adjust the seasoning, if necessary. Serve in a warmed cup with a swirl of the yogurt and a pinch of cumin.

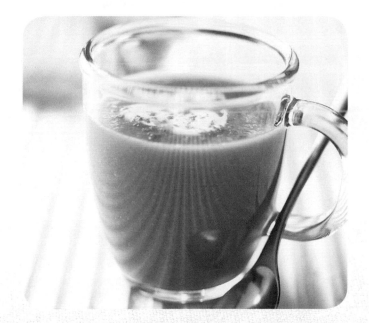

84

GINGER

The plant compounds in fresh ginger have a powerful cancer-destroying action, are anti-inflammatory, can calm nausea, and aid digestion.

For thousands of years, ginger has been considered a healthy food and recent research has borne this out. The main active compounds are terpenes and gingerols, which have anticancer properties and have been shown to destroy colon, ovarian, and rectal cancer cells. Gingerols also have a powerful anti-inflammatory action and ginger has been shown to improve pain and swelling in up to 75 percent of people with arthritis—it also improves mobility. It may also ease migraine tension. Ginger has long been used as a remedy for nausea and to aid digestion, relaxing the intestines, and helping to eliminate flatulence.

- As effective as prescription medicine in beating motion sickness without drowsiness.
- Proven relief from the pain of arthritis.
- Digestive aid.

Practical tips:
Try to buy fresh ginger rather than other forms of ginger, such as ground or preserved, because this contains the highest levels of beneficial compounds. Fresh ginger can be stored in the refrigerator and peeled, chopped, or grated as required. Make a soothing ginger drink by combining freshly grated ginger, lemon juice, honey, and hot water.

DID YOU KNOW?

Ginger is a type of root known as a rhizome and grows underground in tropical climates.

MAJOR NUTRIENTS PER ½ oz/15 g GINGER

Kcalories	19
Total fat	0.3 g
Protein	0.5 g
Carbohydrate	3.8 g
Fiber	0.7 g
Vitamin B1	0.4 mg
Magnesium	10 mg
Potassium	73 mg
Iron	0.6 mg

Carrot and ginger energizer

SERVES 2

generous 1 cup carrot juice

4 tomatoes, peeled, seeded,
    and coarsely chopped

1 tbsp lemon juice

1 oz/25 g fresh parsley

1 tbsp grated fresh ginger

6 ice cubes

½ cup water

chopped fresh parsley, to garnish

Method

1 Place the carrot juice, tomatoes, and lemon juice in a food processor and process gently until combined.

2 Add the parsley to the food processor along with the ginger and ice cubes. Process until well combined, then pour in the water and process until smooth.

3 To serve, pour the mixture into glasses and garnish with chopped fresh parsley.

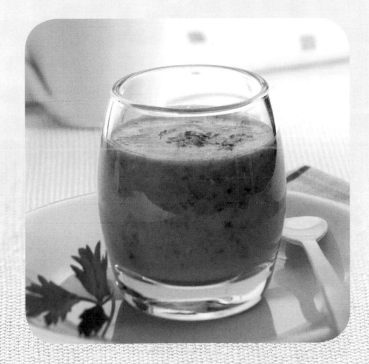

85 NUTMEG

Compounds in nutmeg are sedative, anesthetic, and antibacterial. The fruit also contains monoterpenes, which can help prevent cardiovascular disease.

Nutmeg is actually the fruit from an evergreen native to Indonesia, that is now grown in several countries. The spice is made from the seed of this fruit. The fruit contains the compounds myristicin and elemicin, which are mildly sedative and anesthetic. It also contains monoterpenes, which are believed to have anticoagulant action and may help prevent cardiovascular disease. Like many other spices, nutmeg has antibacterial action and can help to protect us from food poisoning bacteria, such as *E.coli*. Nutmeg has also been used to treat Crohn's disease, an inflammatory condition of the bowel, and it is said that the essential oil of the fruit can help painful gums.

- Mildly sedative.
- Helps prevent blood clots and cardiovascular disease.
- Antibacterial.
- May be anti-inflammatory.

DID YOU KNOW?

Nutmeg is a hallucinogenic and is toxic in large quantities, so use it sparingly. A teaspoonful or less in a recipe will be sufficient.

MAJOR NUTRIENTS PER ½ oz/15 g NUTMEG

Kcalories	12
Total fat	0.8 g
Protein	Trace
Carbohydrate	1 g
Fiber	0.5 g
Magnesium	4 mg
Potassium	8 mg
Calcium	4 mg

Practical tips:
Nutmeg is best used freshly grated from a whole dried fruit—ground nutmeg quickly loses its aroma and flavor. Nutmeg goes well with cooked fruits such as apples and with milk desserts, such as rice pudding. Nutmeg can also be used in savory dishes, such as game casseroles, meat sauces, and curries. A little nutmeg can be stirred into spinach and carrots toward the end of cooking time.

High-fiber nutmeg and cinnamon muffins

MAKES 12

canola oil, for oiling (optional)
5 oz/140 g high-fiber bran cereal
generous 1 cup skim milk
1 cup whole wheat flour
1 tbsp baking powder
½ tsp freshly grated nutmeg
1 tsp ground cinnamon
½ cup light brown sugar
⅔ cup raisins
2 eggs
6 tbsp canola oil

Method

1 Preheat the oven to 400°F/200°C. Oil a 12-hole muffin pan or line with 12 paper cases. Place the cereal and milk in a bowl and let soak for 5 minutes, or until the cereal has softened.

2 Meanwhile, sift the flour, baking powder, nutmeg, and cinnamon together into a large bowl. Stir in the sugar and raisins.

3 Lightly beat the eggs in a large pitcher or bowl, then beat in the oil. Make a well in the center of the dry ingredients and pour in the beaten liquid ingredients and the cereal mixture. Stir gently until just combined; do not overmix.

4 Spoon the batter into the prepared muffin pan. Bake in the preheated oven for about 20 minutes, until well risen, golden brown, and firm to the touch.

5 Leave the muffins in the pan for 5 minutes to cool slightly, then serve warm or transfer to a wire rack and let cool.

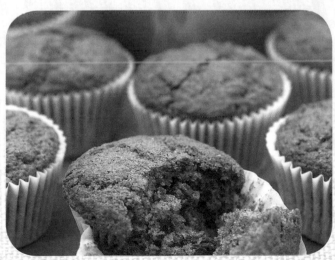

86

TURMERIC

The warm spice turmeric contains healing properties as powerful as modern drugs in the fight against inflammatory diseases such as arthritis.

Turmeric comes from the orange-fleshed root of a plant native to Indonesia and southern India. Its volatile oils and curcumin, the yellow/orange pigment, have been proved to offer protection against inflammatory diseases comparable to modern drugs. Curcumin is thought to be the main health-promoting compound in turmeric, and studies have shown that it is also a powerful antioxidant. Turmeric can help prevent colon cancer and inhibit the growth of certain types of cancer cells, such as breast and prostate cancers. The compound is also able to lower "bad" cholesterol, and increase "good" cholesterol.

- Powerful anti-inflammatory.
- Contains anticancer properties.
- Improves blood cholesterol profile.
- May slow progression of Alzheimer's disease and multiple sclerosis.

DID YOU KNOW?

Turmeric was traditionally called Indian saffron because of its deep yellow color, and has been used throughout history as a textile dye as well as a spice. For this reason it is hard to remove turmeric stains from clothing.

MAJOR NUTRIENTS PER ½ oz/15 G TURMERIC

Kcalories	24
Total fat	0.7 g
Protein	0.5 g
Carbohydrate	4.4 g
Fiber	1.4 g
Folate	225 mcg
Magnesium	13 mg
Potassium	172 mg
Iron	2.8 mg

Practical tips:
You can usually only find ground turmeric in stores. Store it in an airtight container. Make your own curry blend with four parts turmeric, one part chili powder, one part cumin seed, and one part coriander seed. Add a little turmeric to lentils when cooking them, or to yogurt for a healthy dip. Stir-fry vegetables, such as cauliflower or green beans, in oil with turmeric added.

Turmeric yogurt soup

SERVES 4–6

heaping ⅓ cup chickpea flour
1 tsp ground turmeric
¼ tsp chili powder
½ tsp salt, to taste
1¾ cups low-fat plain yogurt
2 tbsp peanut oil
3 cups water

To garnish

½ tbsp peanut oil
¾ tsp cumin seeds
½ tsp black mustard seeds
½ tsp fenugreek seeds
4–6 fresh red chiles, depending
   on how many you are serving

Method

1 Mix the chickpea flour, turmeric, chili powder, and the salt together in a large bowl. Using a whisk or fork, beat in the yogurt until no lumps remain.

2 Heat the oil in a heavy-bottom saucepan over medium–high heat. Mix in the yogurt mixture and then the water, whisking continuously. Bring to a boil, then reduce the heat to very low and simmer, still whisking frequently, for 8 minutes, or until the soup thickens slightly and doesn't have a "raw" taste any longer.

3 Heat the oil for the garnish in a small skillet. Add the cumin, mustard, and fenugreek seeds and stir around until the seeds start to jump and crackle. Add the chiles, remove the skillet from the heat, and stir for about 30 seconds, or until the chiles blister (if the chiles are fresh, they might burst and "jump," so stand well back). Ladle the soup into warmed soup bowls, spoon the fried spices and oil over the top, and serve.

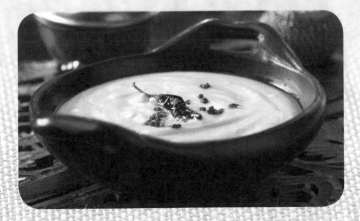

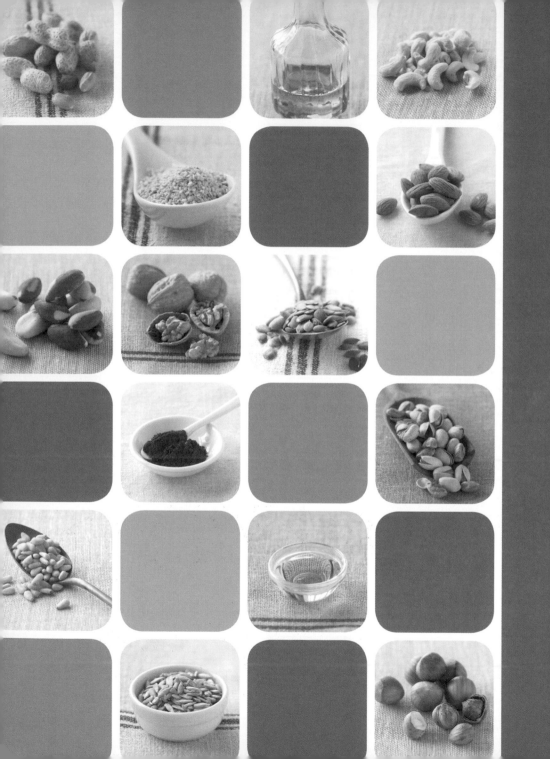

NUTS, SEEDS, AND OILS

High in protein, essential fats, and minerals, nuts, seeds, and oils are a vital part of any diet. Replace nutrient-empty oils with healthier alternatives and eat nuts and seed on their own as a quick snack, in a muesli, or add them to a spicy stir-fry.

(V) Suitable for vegetarians
(D) Ideal for dieters
(P) Suitable for pregnancy
(C) Suitable for children over 5 years
(Q) Quick to prepare and cook

87

PEANUTS

Rich in antioxidants and vitamin E, peanuts can improve blood cholesterol levels and help prevent strokes, heart disease, cancers, and cognitive decline.

Research has found that peanuts rival the antioxidant content of blackberries and strawberries. They are rich in antioxidant polyphenols, including coumaric acid, to help thin the blood, and resveratrol, which can protect against hardened arteries. They have high vitamin E content, an antioxidant linked with heart and arterial health, brain power, and protection from strokes, heart attacks, and cancer. Peanuts contain mostly monounsaturated fat, which has a better effect on blood cholesterol levels than polyunsaturates. They are a good source of the amino acids tryptophan, which helps boost mood, and l-tyrosine, which is linked with brain power.

- Rich in antioxidants, which protect against heart disease.
- High in amino acids to boost mood and brain function.
- Contain phytosterols, which may help prevent colon cancer.
- Rich in monounsaturated fats, which are linked with protection against heart disease.

Practical tips:
Ideally, buy peanuts in their shells, or at least in their skins—they will keep for longer. Fresh peanuts should smell fresh, not musty. Buy unsalted peanuts and store them in a refrigerator—their high oil content means that they don't last long in warm conditions. Make your own healthy peanut butter by blending with a little peanut oil until it has a good spreading consistency.

DID YOU KNOW?
Peanuts, also known as groundnuts, are not in fact true nuts but members of the legume family, like peas or beans.

MAJOR NUTRIENTS PER 1 oz/30 g SHELLED PEANUTS

Kcalories	170
Total fat	14.7 g
Protein	7.7 g
Carbohydrate	4.8 g
Fiber	2.5 g
Niacin	3.6 mg
Folate	72 mcg
Vitamin E	2.5 mg
Calcium	28 mg
Potassium	212 mg
Magnesium	50 mg
Iron	1.4 mg
Zinc	1 mg

Hot and spicy chicken with peanuts

SERVES 4

2 tbsp soy sauce

1 tsp chili powder, or to taste

12 oz/350 g chicken breasts,
  skinned and cut into chunks

5 tbsp peanut oil, plus extra
  if necessary

1 garlic clove, finely chopped

1 tsp grated fresh ginger

3 shallots, thinly sliced

8 oz/225 g carrots, peeled and
  thinly sliced

1 tsp white wine vinegar

pinch of sugar

⅔ cup roasted peanuts

fresh cilantro sprigs, to garnish

boiled rice, to serve

Method

1 Mix the soy sauce and chili powder together in a bowl. Add the chicken chunks and toss to coat. Cover with plastic wrap and let marinate in the refrigerator for 30 minutes.

2 Heat 4 tablespoons of the oil in a skillet. Add the chicken and stir-fry over medium–high heat until browned and well cooked. Remove the chicken from the pan and keep warm.

3 If necessary, add a little more oil to the pan. Add the garlic, ginger, shallots, and carrots and stir-fry for 2–3 minutes.

4 Return the chicken to the pan and stir-fry until it is warmed through again. Add the vinegar, sugar, and peanuts, stir well, and drizzle with the remaining 1 tablespoon of oil. Garnish with cilantro sprigs and serve immediately with cooked rice.

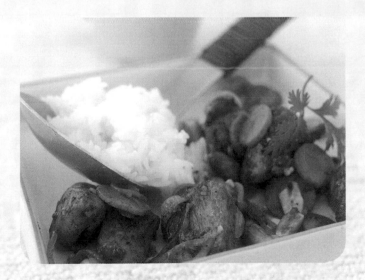

CASHEWS

High in monounsaturated fats, cashews help protect the heart, and contain a range of minerals for strong bones, improved immunity, and increased energy levels.

Cashews are considerably lower in total fat than all other nuts and could be useful as a dieter's snack. Much of this fat is monounsaturated oleic acid (the type found in olive oil), which has health benefits, including protection from heart and arterial disease. Cashews are also rich in important minerals, including magnesium for strong bones and heart health, immune-boosting zinc, and iron for healthy blood and energy. Like other nuts, cashews are linked with protection from cardiovascular disease. People who regularly eat nuts are less likely to die from these diseases than people who never eat nuts.

- Regularly eating nuts is linked with considerably lower risk of dying from cardiovascular diseases.
- Good source of monounsaturated fats linked to protection from disease.
- A good source of B vitamins for brain power and energy.
- Rich in zinc to boost the immune system.

Practical tips:
You can use cashews to make cashew nut butter at home just as you would peanuts (see page 192). Buy whole, shelled cashews and store in the refrigerator. Combine cashews with dried apricots for a healthy mineral-rich snack. Add a handful of cashews to a vegetable stir-fry for a healthy meal.

DID YOU KNOW?
Commercially roasted cashews will have lost the benefit of their unsaturated oils, which are oxidized at high temperatures, but you can roast raw cashews at home in a low-heated oven for 20 minutes.

MAJOR NUTRIENTS PER 1 oz/30 G CASHEWS

Kcalories	166
Total fat	13 g
Protein	5.5 g
Carbohydrate	9 g
Fiber	1 g
Vitamin B1	0.1 mg
Niacin	0.3 mg
Vitamin B6	0.12 mg
Potassium	198 mg
Magnesium	88 mg
Iron	2 mg
Zinc	1.7 mg
Selenium	6 mcg

Sweet-and-sour vegetables with cashews

SERVES 4

1 tbsp peanut oil

1 tsp chili oil

2 onions, sliced

2 carrots, peeled and thinly sliced

2 zucchini, thinly sliced

4 oz/115 g broccoli, cut
into florets

4 oz/115 g button mushrooms,
sliced

4 oz/115 g small bok choy, halved

1 rounded tbsp light brown sugar

2 tbsp light soy sauce

1 tbsp rice vinegar

heaping ⅓ cup toasted cashews

Method

1 Heat both oils in a large skillet. Add the onions and stir-fry over medium heat for 1 2 minutes, or until they start to soften.

2 Add the carrots, zucchini, and broccoli and stir-fry for an additional 2–3 minutes. Add the mushrooms, bok choy, sugar, soy sauce, and vinegar and stir-fry for 1–2 minutes.

3 Sprinkle the toasted cashews over the stir-fry and serve immediately.

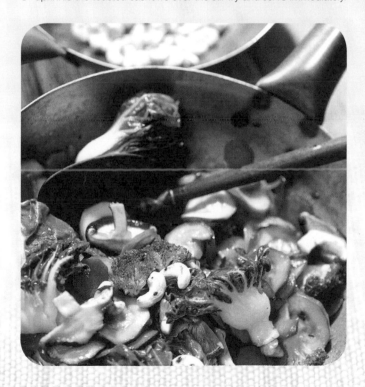

89

ALMONDS

The very high vitamin E content of almonds offers protection against cancer, heart disease, heart attacks and strokes, arthritis, infertility, and skin problems.

Almonds are the seeds of the drupe fruit related to peaches and plums. They are rich in monounsaturated fats and, due to their high fat content, take a long time for the body to digest. This can help keep hunger at bay and help people watching their weight. Almonds are extremely high in vitamin E, which protects against cancer and cardiovascular diseases, helps reduce the pain of osteoarthritis, and keeps skin healthy. Vitamin E can also boost male fertility. Almonds are higher in calcium than almost any other plant food and are therefore an excellent addition to vegan diets and for those who don't eat dairy products.

- Satisfying snack to keep hunger at bay and blood sugar levels even.
- Rich in the antioxidant vitamin E.
- Very good source of calcium.
- High in monounsaturated fat for arterial and heart health.

Practical tips:
Buy whole almonds still in their shells or, at least, still in their brown skins—these keep better than blanched, chopped, or slivered almonds. Store in a cool, dark, dry place—the refrigerator is ideal. Almonds marry very well with apricots, peaches, chicken, rice, and red bell peppers.

DID YOU KNOW?

There is a type of inedible almond, which contains a form of cyanide, known as the bitter almond, that is poisonous but is unavailable in stores.

MAJOR NUTRIENTS PER 1 oz/30 G ALMONDS

Kcalories	174
Total fat	15 g
Protein	6.6 g
Carbohydrate	6 g
Fiber	3 g
Vitamin E	7.4 mg
Niacin	1 mg
Calcium	65 mg
Potassium	206 mg
Magnesium	43 mg
Iron	1 mg
Zinc	1 mcg

Almond and banana smoothie

SERVES 3–4

heaping ¾ cup whole
blanched almonds
2½ cups dairy-free milk
2 ripe bananas, halved
1 tsp natural vanilla extract
ground cinnamon, for dusting

Method

1 Place the almonds in a food processor and process until very finely chopped. Add the milk, bananas, and vanilla extract and blend until smooth and creamy.

2 Pour the mixture into tall glasses, dust with cinnamon, and serve.

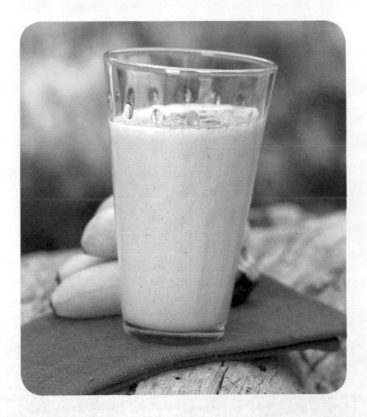

90

BRAZIL NUTS

One of the richest food sources of the antioxidant, anticancer mineral selenium, Brazil nuts are also a good source of calcium and magnesium for healthy bones.

Brazil nuts have a very high total fat content. Much of this is monounsaturated, but there is also a reasonable amount of polyunsaturates and a high content of omega-6 linoleic acid, one of the essential fats. When cooked at high temperatures, these fats oxidize and are no longer healthy, so Brazil nuts are best eaten raw. The nut is extraordinary in its extremely high content of the mineral selenium and, on average, just one to two nuts can provide a whole day's recommended intake. Selenium helps protect us from the diseases of aging. The nuts are also a good source of magnesium and calcium.

- Extremely rich in selenium, a mineral often lacking in modern diets.
- Antioxidant, anti-aging, and anticancer.
- High magnesium content protects heart and bones.
- A good source of vitamin E for healthy skin and healing.

Practical tips:
Keep unshelled nuts in a cool, dry, and dark place for up to six months. The shells of Brazil nuts are tough to crack so purchase a good quality nutcracker. Shelled nuts should be stored in the refrigerator and consumed within a few weeks because their high fat content means they go rancid quickly. They are best eaten raw as a handy snack or added to your breakfast muesli.

DID YOU KNOW?

Brazil nuts are not actually nuts, but seeds that are enclosed in a hard fruit the size of a coconut. The trees grow wild in the Amazon rainforests of Brazil and are rarely successfully cultivated.

MAJOR NUTRIENTS PER 1 oz/30 G BRAZIL NUTS

Kcalories	197
Total fat	19.9 g
Protein	4.3 g
Carbohydrate	3.7 g
Fiber	2.3 g
Vitamin E	1.7 mcg
Calcium	48 mg
Potassium	198 mg
Magnesium	113 mg
Zinc	1.2 mg
Selenium	575 mcg

Trail mix

MAKES 4½ CUPS

½ cup chopped ready-to-eat dried
    apricots
½ cup dried cranberries
½ cup roasted cashews
½ cup shelled hazelnuts
½ cup shelled Brazil nuts, halved
½ cup slivered almonds
4 tbsp toasted pumpkin seeds
4 tbsp sunflower seeds
4 tbsp toasted pine nuts

Method

1 Place all the ingredients in an airtight container, close the lid, and
shake several times. Shake the container before each opening, then
reseal. This mix will stay fresh for up to 2 weeks if tightly sealed after
each opening.

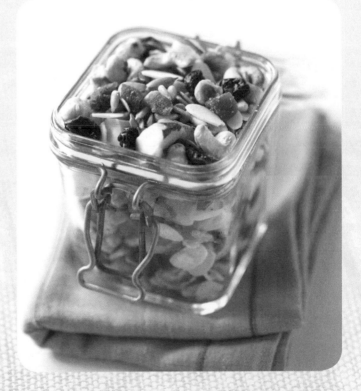

91

WALNUTS

Known for their unusually high content of omega-3 fat, walnuts can help prevent heart disease, cancers, arthritis, skin complaints, and nervous system disorders.

Unlike most nuts, walnuts are much richer in polyunsaturated fats than in monounsaturates. The type of polyunsaturates that walnuts contain is mostly the essential omega-3 fats, in the form of alpha-linolenic acid. Just one 1¼ oz/30 g portion will provide you with more than a day's recommended intake. An adequate and balanced intake of the omega fats has been linked with protection from aging, cardiovascular disease, cancers, arthritis, skin problems, and diseases of the nervous system. For people who don't eat fish and fish oils, an intake of omega-3 fats from other sources, such as walnuts, flaxseeds, and soy, is important.

- Good source of fiber and B vitamins.
- Rich in omega-3 fats and antioxidants for health protection.
- Good source of a range of important minerals.
- Can lower "bad" cholesterol and blood pressure and increase elasticity of the arteries.

Practical tips:
The high levels of polyunsaturated fats mean that walnuts go rancid easily. Buy nuts with their shells on if possible, store in the refrigerator, and consume quickly. Avoid buying chopped walnuts—chopping speeds the oxidation of the nuts. Walnuts are best eaten raw as a snack, in muesli, or sprinkled on yogurt and fruit.

DID YOU KNOW?

The most popular type of walnut for eating is Juglans Regia, the so-called "English walnut." Black-and-white walnuts are also edible, although their shells are hard to crack.

MAJOR NUTRIENTS PER 1 oz/30 G WALNUTS

Kcalories	196
Total fat	19.5 g
Protein	4.5 g
Carbohydrate	4 g
Fiber	2 g
Niacin	0.3 mg
Vitamin B6	0.16 mg
Calcium	29 mg
Potassium	132 mg
Magnesium	47 mg
Iron	0.9 mg
Zinc	0.9 mg

Walnut and seed bread

MAKES 2 LARGE LOAVES

6½ cups whole wheat flour

scant 1 cup strong white flour,
   plus extra for dusting

2 tbsp sesame seeds

2 tbsp sunflower seeds

2 tbsp poppy seeds

1 cup walnuts, chopped

2 tsp salt

½ oz/15 g active dry yeast

2 tbsp olive oil or walnut oil

3 cups lukewarm water

1 tbsp canola oil, for greasing

Method

1 Mix the flours, seeds, walnuts, salt, and yeast together in a large bowl. Add the oil and water and stir well to form a soft dough. Turn out the dough onto a lightly floured surface and knead well for 5–7 minutes, or until smooth and elastic.

2 Return the dough to the bowl, cover with a damp dish towel, and leave in a warm place for 1–1½ hours to rise, or until the dough has doubled in size. Turn the dough out onto a lightly floured surface and knead again for 1 minute.

3 Grease 2 x 2-lb/900-g loaf pans well with oil. Divide the dough in half. Shape one piece the length of the pan and 3 times the width. Fold the dough in 3 lengthwise and place in one of the pans with the join underneath. Repeat with the other piece of dough.

4 Cover and let rise again in a warm place for about 30 minutes, or until the bread is well risen above the pans.

5 Meanwhile, preheat the oven to 450°F/230°C. Bake in the center of the preheated oven for 25–30 minutes, until golden brown and the loaves sound hollow when tapped on the bases with your knuckles. If the loaves are getting too brown during cooking, reduce the temperature to 425°F/220°C. Transfer to a wire rack to cool.

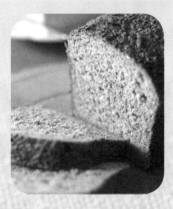

92

PISTACHIOS

Green-tinted pistachios are rich in plant sterols and soluble fibers, which can lower "bad" cholesterol and may protect against cancers.

Pistachios have become widely available in recent years and make a welcome addition to a healthy diet. They are rich in beta-sitosterols, which can help lower "bad" blood cholesterol and may protect against cancer. Pistachios are also a good source of fiber and soluble fiber, which offer benefits for the blood cholesterol profile, and may help prevent certain cancers and symptoms of digestive problems, such as constipation and irritable bowel syndrome. The nuts also contain a range of minerals, B vitamins, and are a good source of protein, being less high in fat than other types of nuts.

- High in sterols, which lower blood cholesterol and may protect against cancer.
- Rich in potassium to lower blood pressure and eliminate fluid.
- High in fiber and soluble fiber to aid the digestive system and improve blood cholesterol profile.
- Help control blood sugar levels and may be of help to diabetics and people who are insulin resistant.

Practical tips:
A dish of unshelled pistachios makes a healthy predinner snack. They are easy to shell before eating and you can eat the brown skin on the nuts, which adds extra fiber and nutrients. Add pistachios to grain salads, breakfast cereals, and stuffings.

DID YOU KNOW?
Pistachios are one of the few nuts to contain carotenes, which cause their distinctive green-colored flesh.

MAJOR NUTRIENTS PER 1 oz/30 g PISTACHIOS

Kcalories	167
Total fat	13.5 g
Protein	6 g
Carbohydrate	8.5 g
Fiber	3 g
Niacin	0.4 mg
Vitamin B6	0.5 mg
Calcium	32 mg
Potassium	308 mg
Magnesium	36 mg
Iron	1.2 mg
Zinc	0.7 mg
Beta-carotene	100 mcg

Chicken with pistachios

SERVES 4

¼ cup chicken stock

2 tbsp light soy sauce

2 tbsp dry sherry

3 tsp cornstarch

1 egg white, beaten

pinch of salt

3 tbsp peanut oil, plus extra if
   necessary

1 lb/450 g skinless chicken breast,
   cut into strips

1 lb/450 g mushrooms, thinly sliced

1 head broccoli, cut into florets

5½ oz/150 g bean sprouts

3½ oz/100 g canned water
   chestnuts, drained and
   thinly sliced

heaping 1 cup pistachios, plus
   extra 1 tbsp to garnish

boiled rice, to serve

Method

1 Mix the chicken stock, soy sauce, sherry, and 1 teaspoon of the cornstarch together in a bowl. Set aside.

2 Mix the egg white, salt, 2 tablespoons of the oil, and 2 teaspoons of the cornstarch together in a large bowl. Add the chicken and toss to coat.

3 Heat a large wok over high heat for 30 seconds. Add the remaining oil, swirl it around to coat the bottom, and heat for 30 seconds. Add the chicken in batches and stir fry until golden. Remove the chicken from the wok, drain on paper towels, and keep warm.

4 Add more oil to the wok if needed and stir-fry the mushrooms, then add the broccoli and stir-fry for an additional 2–3 minutes.

5 Return the chicken to the wok and add the bean sprouts, water chestnuts, and pistachios. Stir-fry until all the ingredients are thoroughly warm. Add the chicken stock mixture and cook, stirring, until thickened. Serve over a bed of rice, garnished with the reserved pistachios.

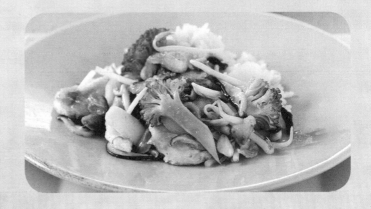

93 PINE NUTS

A source of omega-3 fats for a variety of health benefits, pine nuts are also rich in vitamin E, zinc, and cholesterol-lowering plant sterols.

Pine nuts come from several species of pine tree. All have similar nutritional benefits, although the longer Asian types contain more oil. They are rich in polyunsaturated fat omega-6s, but also contain some of the less widely available omega-3s that are important for heart health as well as brain power. Pine nuts are very rich in Vitamin E and zinc, two antioxidants that help the heart, boost the immune system, and increase fertility. They also contain sterols and stanols, compounds that help lower blood cholesterol.

- High in omega-6 fats and contain omega-3s.
- Contain plant sterols for cholesterol lowering and a healthy immune system.
- Rich in zinc and vitamin E.
- Good source of a range of minerals and fiber.

Practical tips:
Pine nuts have a rich and yet delicate flavor with a hint of resin. They tend to go rancid quickly so buy in small quantities, store in a refrigerator, and use within a few weeks. Pine nuts go well with spinach, strong cheeses, golden raisins, and oily fish. You can make a basil pesto with fresh basil, pine nuts, Parmesan, and olive oil. Lightly dry-fry the nuts to make toasted pine nuts, but do not overcook as they can burn easily and oxidize. Pine nuts are best eaten raw.

DID YOU KNOW?

Research shows that pine nuts have been used for food since the Paleolithic period, which ended around 40,000 years ago.

MAJOR NUTRIENTS PER ½ oz/15 g PINE NUTS

Kcalories	101
Total fat	10 g
Protein	2 g
Carbohydrate	2 g
Fiber	0.6 g
Vitamin E	1.4 mcg
Potassium	90 mg
Magnesium	38 mg
Iron	0.8 mg
Zinc	1 mg

Toasted pine nut and vegetable couscous

SERVES 4

¾ cup dried green lentils

½ cup pine nuts

1 tbsp olive oil

1 onion, diced

2 garlic cloves, crushed

10 oz/280 g zucchini, sliced

9 oz/250 g tomatoes, chopped

14 oz/400 g canned artichoke
  hearts, drained and cut in half
  lengthwise

1¼ cups couscous

2 cups vegetable stock

3 tbsp torn fresh basil leaves, plus
  extra leaves to garnish

pepper

Method

1 Place the lentils in a saucepan with plenty of cold water. Bring to a boil and boil rapidly for 10 minutes. Reduce the heat, cover, and simmer for 15 minutes, or until tender.

2 Meanwhile, heat a nonstick skillet over medium heat. Add the pine nuts and lightly toast, shaking the skillet frequently, for 3–4 minutes, or until golden brown. Tip into a small bowl and set aside.

3 Heat the oil in a nonstick skillet over medium heat. Add the onion, garlic, and zucchini and cook, stirring frequently, for 8–10 minutes, or until tender and the zucchini have browned slightly. Add the tomatoes and artichoke halves and heat through thoroughly for 5 minutes.

4 Meanwhile, place the couscous in a heatproof bowl. Bring the stock to a boil in a saucepan. Pour over the couscous, cover, and leave for 10 minutes, until the couscous absorbs the stock and becomes tender.

5 Drain the lentils and stir into the couscous. Stir in the torn basil and season well with pepper. Transfer the couscous to a warmed serving dish and spoon over the cooked vegetables. Sprinkle the toasted pine nuts over the top, garnish with basil leaves, and serve immediately.

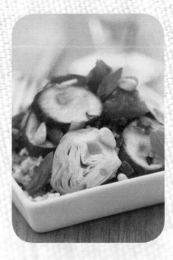

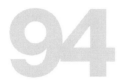

HAZELNUTS

Particularly rich in potassium, hazelnuts have the ability to reduce fluid retention and lower blood pressure.

Hazelnuts are a good source of protein and monounsaturated fats, which have been shown to reduce "bad" cholesterol in the blood and even slightly raise "good" cholesterol. The nuts are high in beta-sitosterol, a plant fat that can help reduce an enlarged prostate and is also a cholesterol-lowering compound. Hazelnuts are very high in vitamin E, an antioxidant that maintains skin health, heart health, and which can boost the immune system. The high potassium content can help people with high blood pressure and is also a diuretic. The magnesium content helps heart health and can contribute to bone strength.

- High in beta-sitosterol, which may help prostate health.
- Rich in monounsaturates, which can help improve blood cholesterol profile.
- Very rich in antioxidant vitamin E.
- Good source of soluble fiber for lowering "bad" cholesterol and digestive health.

Practical tips:
Hazelnuts keep better than many other nuts because they contain less fat and their vitamin E acts as a preservative. Buy whole nuts rather than chopped—this destroys much of their nutrient content. Store in a refrigerator. Use as a snack, or add to salads, stir-fries, breakfast cereals, and desserts.

DID YOU KNOW?
Hazelnuts are also known as filberts or cobnuts, depending on their country of origin.

MAJOR NUTRIENTS PER 1 oz/30 G HAZELNUTS

Kcalories	188
Total fat	18.2 g
Protein	4.5 g
Carbohydrate	5 g
Fiber	2.9 g
Vitamin E	4.5 mg
Niacin	0.5 mg
Vitamin B6	0.16 mg
Folate	34 mcg
Potassium	204 mg
Magnesium	49 mg
Iron	1.4 mg
Zinc	0.7 mg

Vegetable and hazelnut loaf

MAKES 1 LOAF

2 tbsp canola oil, plus extra
    for oiling
1 onion, chopped
1 garlic clove, finely chopped
2 celery stalks, chopped
1 tbsp all-purpose flour
7 fl oz/200 ml strained canned
    tomatoes
2 cups fresh whole wheat
    breadcrumbs
2 carrots, peeled and grated
¾ cup toasted hazelnuts, ground
1 tbsp dark soy sauce
2 tbsp chopped fresh cilantro
1 egg, lightly beaten
salt and pepper
mixed red and green lettuce leaves,
    to serve

Method

1 Preheat the oven to
   350°F/180°C. Oil and line a
   1-lb/450-g loaf pan. Heat the
   oil in a heavy-bottom skillet.
   Add the onion and cook over
   medium heat, stirring
   frequently, for 5 minutes, or
   until softened. Add the garlic
   and celery and cook, stirring
   frequently, for 5 minutes. Add
   the flour and cook, stirring, for
   1 minute. Gradually stir in the
   strained canned tomatoes and
   cook, stirring continuously,
   until thickened. Remove the
   skillet from the heat.

2 Place the breadcrumbs,
   carrots, ground hazelnuts, soy
   sauce, and cilantro in a bowl.
   Add the tomato mixture and
   stir well. Cool slightly, then
   beat in the egg and season
   with salt and pepper.

3 Spoon the mixture into the
   prepared pan and smooth the
   surface. Cover with aluminum
   foil and bake in the preheated
   oven for 1 hour. If serving hot,
   turn the loaf out onto a warmed
   serving dish and serve with
   lettuce. Alternatively, cool the loaf
   in the pan before turning out.

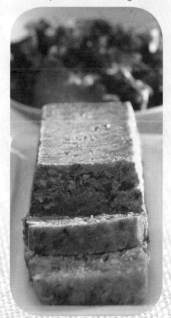

95

SESAME SEEDS

The lignan fibers in sesame seeds help lower "bad" cholesterol, and the seeds may also have an anti-inflammatory action, reducing the pain of arthritis.

Sesame seeds contain two special types of fiber—sesamin and sesamolin—which are members of the lignans group. They can lower "bad" cholesterol and help prevent high blood pressure which helps to protect against cardiovascular disease. Sesamin is a powerful antioxidant in its own right and has been shown to protect the liver from damage. Plant sterols contained in the seeds also have a cholesterol-lowering action. The seeds are particularly rich in copper, which may be of use to arthritis sufferers because it is thought to have an anti-inflammatory action, reducing pain and swelling. Sesame seeds also contain the minerals iron, zinc, calcium, and potassium in varying quantities.

- Good source of plant fibers and sterols to help lower cholesterol.
- Source of the antioxidant lignan sesamin.
- High in iron and zinc.
- Contain large amounts of calcium useful for non-dairy eaters.

Practical tips:
Store in a cool, dry, dark place in an airtight tin. Sesame seeds can be eaten raw or lightly toasted in an oven on low heat, but do not overcook—this destroys some healthy fats. Sprinkle the seeds on vegetables such as broccoli or spinach before serving, or add to grain salads. Sesame seed oil is good for stir-fries while tahini, a sesame seed paste, can be added to hummus and other dips.

DID YOU KNOW?

Sesame seeds can be found in a range of colors that include pale cream, brown, red, and black; the darker the color, the stronger the flavor tends to be.

MAJOR NUTRIENTS PER ½ oz/15 G SESAME SEEDS

Kcalories	85
Total fat	7.2 g
Protein	2.5 g
Carbohydrate	3.9 g
Fiber	2.5 g
Niacin	0.8 mg
Folate	14 mcg
Calcium	20 mg
Potassium	61 mg
Magnesium	52 mg
Iron	1.2 mg
Zinc	1.5 mg

Snow pea, sesame seed, and tofu stir-fry

SERVES 2–3

1 tbsp toasted sesame oil

2 tbsp peanut oil

7 oz/200 g small shiitake
　mushrooms

2 heads bok choy, leaves left
　whole, stalks sliced

5½ oz/150 g snow peas, sliced
　in half at an angle

9 oz/250 g firm tofu, cut into cubes

1¼-inch/3-cm piece fresh ginger,
　peeled and thinly sliced

2 garlic cloves, finely chopped

1 tbsp light soy sauce

1 tsp sesame seeds

pepper

cooked noodles, to serve

Method

1 Heat a large wok over high heat for 30 seconds. Add the oils, swirl
them around to coat the bottom, and heat for an additional 30
seconds. Add the mushrooms, bok choy stalks, and snow peas
and stir-fry for 1 minute.

2 Add the tofu, bok choy leaves, ginger, garlic, and a splash of water
and stir-fry for 1–2 minutes, until the bok choy has wilted.

3 Stir in the soy sauce, sprinkle with sesame seeds, and season
with pepper. Serve immediately with cooked noodles.

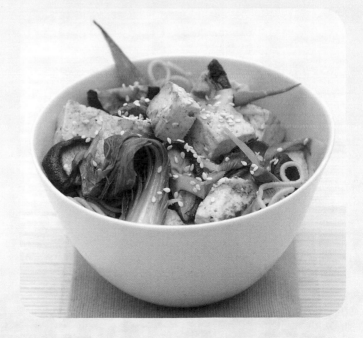

96

PUMPKIN SEEDS

Rich in zinc, pumpkin seeds help boost the immune system and fertility. They also contain sterols linked with protection against hormone-based cancers.

Pumpkin seeds are a nutritious snack and, even in small servings they provide a significant amount of minerals, especially zinc and iron. Zinc is an antioxidant mineral, which boosts the immune system and, for men, improves fertility and protects against prostate enlargement and cancer. Iron is important for healthy blood cells and energy levels. High iron and zinc contents make pumpkin seeds a particularly significant food for vegetarians. The seeds contain sterols, which can help remove "bad" cholesterol from the body as well as helping to inhibit the development of breast, colon, and prostate cancer cells. In addition, pumpkin seeds contain some omega-3 fats, vitamin E, folate, and magnesium that can help maintain heart health.

- Rich in zinc for fertility, immune boosting, and cancer protection.
- Rich in iron for healthy blood and to fight fatigue.
- Can help improve blood cholesterol profile.
- Good source of heart-healthy and anti-inflammatory nutrients.

Practical tips:
Pumpkin seeds are not edible when raw and those for sale are almost always roasted. Chew the seeds well to ensure maximum absorption of nutrients. Add to salads and muesli, or sprinkle on breakfast cereal or yogurt. The seeds can be ground and added to vegetable, nut, and bean burgers.

....

DID YOU KNOW?

If you grow or buy pumpkins and squashes, don't discard the seeds—make your own roasted pumpkin seeds. Wash and dry the seeds and toss in a little groundnut or light olive oil. Spread on a baking sheet and lightly roast on a low heat for 20 minutes.

....

MAJOR NUTRIENTS PER ½ oz/15 g PUMPKIN SEEDS

Kcalories	81
Total fat	6.9 g
Protein	3.7 g
Carbohydrate	2.7 g
Fiber	0.6 g
Niacin	0.3 mg
Potassium	121 mg
Magnesium	80 mg
Iron	2.2 mg
Zinc	1.1 mg

Apple and seed muesli

MAKES 7 CUPS (V) (D) (P) (C) (Q)

⅓ cup sunflower seeds

¼ cup pumpkin seeds

⅔ cup shelled hazelnuts, coarsely
   chopped

4½ oz/125 g buckwheat flakes

4½ oz/125 g rice flakes

4½ oz/125 g millet flakes

4 oz/115 g no-soak dried apple,
   coarsely chopped

4 oz/115 g dried pitted dates,
   coarsely chopped

Method

1 Heat a nonstick skillet over medium heat. Add the seeds and
hazelnuts and lightly toast, shaking the skillet frequently, for 4
minutes, or until golden brown. Transfer to a large bowl and let cool.

2 Add the flakes, apple, and dates to the bowl and mix thoroughly
until combined. Store the muesli in an airtight jar or container.

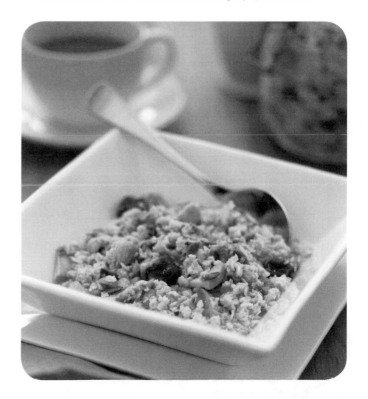

97

SUNFLOWER SEEDS

Rich in a range of minerals and vitamin E, sunflower seeds also offer protection from inflammation and cardiovascular disease.

DID YOU KNOW?

Native to Central and South America, sunflower seeds have been eaten in North America for around 5,000 years, but are now grown all across the world for their high oil content.

MAJOR NUTRIENTS PER ½ oz/15 G SUNFLOWER SEEDS

Kcalories	86
Total fat	7.4 g
Protein	3.4 g
Vitamin E	5 mg
Fiber	1.6 g
Niacin	0.7 mg
Folate	34 mcg
Calcium	17 mg
Potassium	103 mg
Magnesium	53 mg
Selenium	9 mcg
Iron	1 mg
Zinc	0.8 mg

Sunflower seeds, usually sold shelled, are one of the world's major sources of vegetable oil and are rich in polyunsaturated fats. The seeds are also very rich in vitamin E, and can help protect us from inflammatory conditions, such as asthma and rheumatoid arthritis. Vitamin E is also an antioxidant, neutralizing the free radicals that in excess can damage the body cells and speed up the aging process. It is also linked with a lower risk of cardiovascular disease and with protection from colon cancer. Sunflower seeds are rich in plant sterols, which have a cholesterol-lowering effect, and various minerals including iron, magnesium, and selenium.

- Rich in the omega-6 linoleic acid, which is an essential fat.
- Very high in antioxidant vitamin E, which has a range of health benefits.
- High in plant sterols for cholesterol-lowering effect.
- Nutrient and mineral rich.

Practical tips:
The high polyunsaturated content of sunflower seeds means that they spoil quickly and can go rancid if kept in warm conditions. Shelled nuts and seeds can be frozen and thawed at room temperature. The seeds make a good addition to salads, muesli, and oatmeal, or can be eaten as a snack.

Sunflower seed muffins

MAKES 12

6 tbsp canola oil, plus extra for
  oiling (optional)

1 cup whole wheat flour

1 tbsp baking powder

½ cup light brown sugar

scant 2 cups rolled oats

heaping ½ cup golden raisins

heaping ½ cup sunflower seeds

2 eggs

generous 1 cup skim milk

1 tsp vanilla extract

Method

1 Preheat the oven to 400°F/200°C. Oil a 12-hole muffin pan or line with 12 paper cases. Sift together the flour and baking powder into a large bowl, adding the contents of the strainer back into the bowl. Stir in the sugar, oats, golden raisins, and scant ½ cup of the sunflower seeds.

2 Lightly beat the eggs in a large pitcher or bowl, then beat in the milk, oil, and vanilla extract. Make a well in the center of the dry ingredients and pour in the beaten liquid ingredients. Stir gently until just combined; do not overmix.

3 Spoon the batter into the prepared muffin pan. Sprinkle the remaining sunflower seeds over the tops of the muffins. Bake in the preheated oven for about 20 minutes, until well risen, golden brown, and firm to the touch.

4 Leave the muffins in the pan for 5 minutes to cool slightly, then serve warm or transfer to a wire rack and let cool.

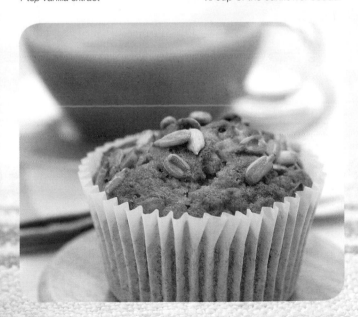

CHOCOLATE AND COCOA POWDER

98

Not just an indulgent treat, the cocoa bean contains flavonoids, magnesium, and iron for protection from heart disease.

Chocolate is made from cocoa beans, which are rich in antioxidant flavonoids, fiber, and minerals. The chocolate-making process also provides procyanidins, which have an anti-inflammatory action. For better or worse, chocolate contains caffeine and a 3½ oz/100 g bar of dark chocolate has about as much as a cup of coffee. Cocoa powder is a relatively low-fat, high fiber source of minerals and antioxidants and for chocolate lovers watching their fat intake, a cocoa drink made with skim milk is a good alternative.

- Antioxidant content can have an anticoagulant action and protect against the oxidation of cholesterol in our bodies.
- Magnesium content protects the heart.
- Iron content can keep blood healthy and maintain energy levels.
- Contains the stimulant theobromine, which is a diuretic.

Practical tips:
The type of chocolate that we buy has a strong bearing on the amount of nutrients it contains. Generally, the more cocoa solids that the chocolate contains, the more antioxidants and minerals it has. This means that dark chocolate with 70 percent cocoa solids is a good source, while standard milk chocolate is not. Cocoa butter is high in total fat and saturated fat, so even dark chocolate should be consumed in moderate amounts. White chocolate is a mix of cocoa butter and milk solids and has negligible healthy nutrients.

DID YOU KNOW?
Cocoa beans grow on cocoa trees that are now mainly grown in South America and Africa. They were first imported to Europe by Christopher Columbus in the early 16th century.

MAJOR NUTRIENTS PER ½ oz/15 G COCOA POWDER

Kcalories	34
Total fat	2 g
Protein	3 g
Carbohydrate	8 g
Fiber	5 g
Calcium	19 mg
Magnesium	22 mg
Potassium	229 mg
Iron	2 mg
Zinc	1 mg

Chicken with chile and chocolate

SERVES 6–8

1 whole garlic bulb

1 chicken, weighing 4 lb 8 oz/2 kg

4 fresh mint sprigs

½ tsp black peppercorns

2–3 cloves

salt

warm cornmeal tortillas and
   guacamole, to serve

Sauce

3–4 tbsp olive oil

1 large onion, finely sliced

1 red bell pepper, seeded and
   diced

1 lb 2 oz/500 g fresh or canned
   tomatoes, peeled and chopped

1 ripe plantain or unripe banana,
   peeled and cut into chunks

⅔ cup blanched almonds,
   toasted and crushed

1 tsp cumin seeds

1 tsp allspice berries

1 soft cornmeal tortilla, torn into
   pieces, or 1 tbsp tortilla chips

1¾ oz/50 g dried chiles, seeded,
   soaked in boiling water for
   20 minutes, and drained

2 tbsp raisins

finely grated rind of 1 orange

2 tbsp cocoa powder or
   1¾ oz/50 g good-quality
   semisweet chocolate

Method

1 Preheat the oven to 350°F/180°C. Score around the center of the garlic bulb. Cut the chicken into 12 pieces, rinse, and place in a large saucepan with enough cold water to cover. Bring to a boil, skimming off any foam, then add the garlic, mint, peppercorns, cloves, and a little salt. Return to a boil, then reduce the heat, cover, and simmer for 30–40 minutes, until the chicken is tender. Transfer to an ovenproof dish. Strain the stock and set aside.

2 To make the sauce, heat 2 tablespoons of the oil in a skillet. Add the onion and cook over low heat for 10–15 minutes. Remove with a slotted spoon and set aside. Reheat the oily juices in the pan, add the bell pepper, and cook for 5–6 minutes. Add the tomatoes and plantain and heat until bubbling, then reduce the heat, cover, and cook over low heat for 20 minutes, until the plantain is tender.

3 Heat a nonstick skillet over medium–high heat. Add the almonds and spices to toast, shake the skillet frequently until golden. Transfer to a food processor and pulse. Set aside.

4 Tip the onion and tomato mixture into a food processor. Add the tortilla, chiles, and soaking water and process until smooth. You may need to add a little of the chicken stock.

5 Add the remaining oil to the skillet and reheat. Add the crushed nuts and spices and stir-fry for 1–2 minutes. Add the tomato mixture and heat until bubbling, reduce the heat and cook for 5 minutes. Add the raisins, orange rind, and 4 cups of the stock. Bring to a boil, reduce the heat, and simmer for 20 minutes, until the liquid is reduced by a third. Stir in the cocoa and heat gently.

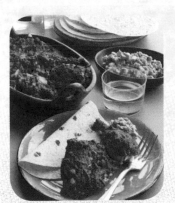

6 Pour the sauce over the chicken in the dish, cover, and cook in the preheated oven for 20–25 minutes. Serve with warm tortillas and guacamole.

99

OLIVE OIL

Well known for being high in heart protective monounsaturates, virgin olive oils also contain a range of antioxidant plant compounds and vitamin E.

The main type of fat in olive oil is monounsaturated, which helps prevent cholesterol being deposited on artery walls and therefore helps protect us from cardiovascular disease and strokes. In addition, early pressings of the olives (as in extra virgin olive oil, particularly "cold pressed" oil) produce an oil that is rich in beneficial plant compounds. These can protect against cancer and high blood pressure, lower cholesterol, and the particular compound oleocanthal, an anti-inflammatory with similar action to ibuprofen. Finally, olive oil is a good source of vitamin E.

- Helps improve blood cholesterol profile and protect us from cardiovascular disease.
- Rich in polyphenols to protect against colon and other cancers.
- Can help prevent *H.pylori* which can lead to stomach ulcers.
- Antibacterial and antioxidant.

Practical tips:
Olive oil should be stored in the dark and used within one to two months. When buying olive oil, choose a store that keeps it in dimly lit conditions and has a high turnover. For the full benefit of olive oil, eat it cold in salad dressings or drizzled on bread or vegetables. Don't use extra virgin olive oil for cooking at high temperatures or the beneficial chemicals will be destroyed.

DID YOU KNOW?
Researchers in Italy have found that light destroys many of the disease-fighting compounds in olive oil. Studies showed that after a year, oils stored in clear bottles under store lighting showed at least a 30 percent decrease in antioxidants.

MAJOR NUTRIENTS PER 1 TBSP/15 ML OLIVE OIL

Kcalories	130
Total fat	15 g
Vitamin E	2.1 g

Lemon pepper olive oil

MAKES GENEROUS 1 CUP

zest of 1 lemon
1 whole lemon
2 tsp multicolored peppercorns
generous 1 cup olive oil

Method

1 Prepare a double boiler. Bring the water in the bottom pan to a boil, reduce the heat, and simmer.

2 Cut the lemon zest into thin strips, making sure you omit the white pith. Thinly slice the other lemon. Crush the peppercorns in a mortar with a pestle. Place the strips of lemon zest, lemon slices, peppercorns, and oil in the top of the double boiler. Cover and cook over simmering water for 1 hour. If you have a digital thermometer, test the oil. It should reach a temperature of 250°F/120°C before you remove it from the double boiler. Make sure you don't let the oil burn.

3 Remove from the heat, let cool, and then strain through cheesecloth into a clean jar. Cover and store in the refrigerator. You can also leave the lemon strips and pepper in the jar and store in the refrigerator, and then strain before using. Brush over white fish fillets or chicken breasts before cooking.

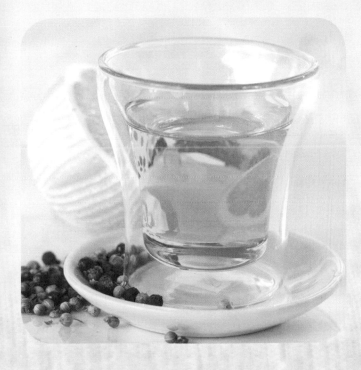

100 CANOLA OIL

This is one of the healthiest oils, rich in monounsaturates and omega-3 fats to protect against cancers, heart disease, and other ailments.

Canola oil had been neglected as a health-giving oil until recently, when more European farmers began producing it as a competitively priced alternative to olive oil. In fact, canola oil in many ways has an even better "health profile" than its rival does. It has nearly as high a content of monounsaturated fat as olive oil and contains higher amounts of the essential omega-3 fat alpha-linoleic acid than any other oil used in quantity for culinary purpose. Canola oil also has a perfect balance between omega-6 and omega-3s and is lower in saturated fat than all the other commonly used oils. It is also a good source of vitamin E.

- Excellent balance of essential fats in line with recommended guidelines.
- Low in saturated fat.
- Good source of the antioxidant vitamin E.
- High in omega-3 fats, which have a variety of health benefits when eaten regularly.

Practical tips:
Refined canola oil is a good choice for cooking because it doesn't degrade when heated. Cold pressed or extra virgin canola oil is a great choice for salad dressings and drizzling. Its nutty flavor is particularly good drizzled over artichoke hearts or asparagus. It is ideal for mayonnaise because it has a milder flavor than olive oil.

DID YOU KNOW?
Canola oil is an annual plant and a member of the brassica family. It has bright yellow flowers in summer and turns many fields golden.

MAJOR NUTRIENTS PER 1 TBSP/15 ML CANOLA OIL

Kcalories	130
Total fat	15 g
Vitamin E	2.6 mg

Garlic, chile, and oregano canola oil

MAKES 1 CUP

5 garlic cloves
2 tbsp red chile
1 tsp dried oregano
generous 1 cup canola oil

Method

1 Preheat the oven to 300°F/150°C.

2 Cut the garlic cloves in half lengthwise. Using gloves, remove the seeds from the chile and chop the flesh into small pieces equalling 2 tablespoons.

3 Mix the garlic, chile, oregano, and oil together in an ovenproof glass dish. Place in the center of the preheated oven and heat for 1½–2 hours. If you have a digital thermometer, test the oil. It should reach a temperature of 250°F/120°C before you remove it from the oven.

4 Remove from the oven, let cool, and then strain through cheesecloth into a clean jar. Cover and store in the refrigerator.

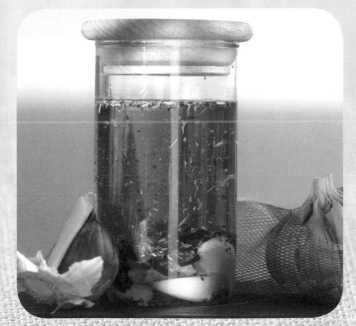

GLOSSARY

Alpha-linolenic acid Type of omega-3 polyunsaturated fat. One of the essential fatty acids we need in small amounts for health because our bodies can't manufacture it.

Amino acids The 22 "building blocks" of protein which are contained in protein foods in varying combinations and amounts. Only 8 of the 22 amino acids are essential in our diet and can only be found in food.

Anthocyanin A purple, red, or blue pigment occuring in certain foods—a powerful antioxidant.

Antioxidant Substance that protects the body against the effects of free radicals, toxins, and pollutants.

Antioxidant scale *See* ORAC.

"Bad" cholesterol/LDL Low-density lipoproteins that transport fats such as cholesterol in the blood. High levels of "bad" cholesterol are linked with the formation of plaques (furring of the arteries) and cardiovascular disease.

Beta-carotene *See* carotenes.

Beta-cryptoxanthin/ cryptoxanthin Strong antioxidant with a particular effect on reducing the risk of certain cancers.

Beta-glucans A type of soluble fiber found in certain plants, including whole grain barley and oats.

Beta-sitosterol A plant sterol, found in certain nuts, seeds, and other plants, which can reduce blood cholesterol.

Bioflavonoid/flavonoid A group of several thousand antioxidant compounds found in fruits, vegetables, and other plant foods.

Carotenes/carotenoids Yellow/ red/orange pigments, found in a variety of plant foods such as carrots, which have several health benefits. The main types are alpha-carotene and beta-carotene. Lutein, lycopene, and zeaxanthin are others.

Catechin A compound from the flavonoid group, found in tea and certain other plants, which can help protect against cardiovascular disease and has other health benefits.

Cholesterol A fatty substance present in many foods of animal origin and manufactured in the liver in humans. It is essential in the body, but under certain circumstances can also encourage the development of coronary artery disease. See "good" and "bad" cholesterols.

Daidzein A plant isoflavone that has mild estrogen-like effects.

DHA Docosahexaenoic acid—a "long chain" omega-3 fatty acid found in oily fish with several health benefits.

Ellagic acid A polyphenol antioxidant with good anticancer properties present in many red fruits/berries and in some nuts.

EPA Eicosapentaenoic acid—a "long chain" omega-3 fatty acid found in oily fish with several health benefits.

Essential fatty acid/essential fat/EFA Essential fats that our bodies need for health, which must be provided in the diet.

Estrogen A hormone produced in women by the ovaries. After menopause, estrogen levels decline sharply and this decline is linked with health problems, including osteoporosis.

Free radical Highly reactive, unstable atoms or molecules in the body, which are a normal by-product of metabolism, and which are believed, in excess, to be a factor in onset of disease and the aging process.

Genistein *See* daidzein.

Glycemic index (GI) A system of ranking carbohydrate foods according to their effect on blood sugar levels.

"Good" cholesterol/HDL High-density lipoproteins that bind to cholesterol and carry it through the blood. They keep the arteries clear and protect against cardiovascular disease.

Homocysteine An amino acid that is synthesized in our bodies. High levels in the blood are a strong risk factor for cardiovascular disease.

Immune system Processes within our bodies that protect against disease and other potentially harmful pathogens.

Indoles Plant compounds found in cabbage and other green vegetables which have strong anticancer activity.

Insoluble fiber This consists mainly of cellulose, and is the indigestible portion of plant foods which moves right though the digestive system, absorbing water, increasing stool bulk, and helping satiety. It can help prevent disorders of the bowel.

Insulin A hormone produced by the pancreas which regulates blood sugar levels.

Inulin A type of carbohydrate which acts as dietary fiber and a prebiotic in our digestive systems and is found in foods such as some root vegetables, chicory, and onions.

Lignan A type of plant estrogen found in some seeds, grains, fruits, and vegetables.

L-tyrosine/tyrosine An amino acid which can help improve brain function and energy levels. It can be found in a variety of high-protein foods.

Lutein *See* carotenes.

Lycopene A type of carotene found in orange/red fruit and vegetables, such as tomatoes, which can help prevent prostate cancer.

Metabolism Chemical changes in the body during which food and drink are broken down.

Monounsaturated fatty acids/fats A type of fat found in most foods, but when found in high quantities such as in olive oil, avocados, and some nuts, it has a beneficial effect on cholesterol levels, cardiovascular disease, and other health problems.

Omega-3 Types of polyunsaturated fat that are vital for normal body functioning. It has a range of health benefits and protects against a variety of diseases.

ORAC The Oxygen Radical Absorbance Capacity, which is an international method of measuring the antioxidant effect of plant foods, according to their capacity to neutralize free radicals.

Pathogen A biological agent that causes disease or illness to its host.

Pectin A type of soluble fiber contained in good amounts in citrus fruits and apples. Its health benefits include a reduction in blood "bad" cholesterol levels.

Phenolic compound/phenol Group of antioxidant plant compounds, including resveratrol, found in grapes.

Phytochemical/phytonutrient Chemical compounds, found in plants, which are known to have benefits to human health, but which are different from vitamins and minerals.

Polyphenol A group of plant chemicals that includes bioflavonoids, phenols, quercetin, and tannins.

Polyunsaturated Type of fat, found in large amounts in most varieties of plant oil, usually high in omega-6 fatty acids.

Prebiotics Compounds, found in several foods, which stimulate the growth of beneficial bacteria in the intestines.

Probiotics "Friendly" gut bacteria that help to boost the immune system and have various other health benefits.

Quercetin An antioxidant found in tea, onions, and apples.

Saponins Plant compounds that have been shown to inhibit tumor growth, and are found in pulses and some other foods.

Soluble fiber A type of fiber found in oats, certain fruits, and vegetables—can have a beneficial effect on digestive health and cholesterol levels.

Sterols/plant sterols/phytosterols A group of plant compounds that can have a cholesterol-lowering effect in the body.

Sulphides/organosulphides Antioxidant and immune-stimulating compounds found in foods such as onions and garlic.

Sulphoraphane A plant compound, found in brassicas such as sprouts, which has anticancer and antidiabeteic properties.

Tannins Plant compounds from the polyphenol group, found in foods such as tea, wine, and pulses, which can inhibit the absorption of minerals but have some health protection effects.

Tryptophan An amino acid that helps to promote relaxation and improve mood.

Zeaxanthin *See* carotenes.

INDEX